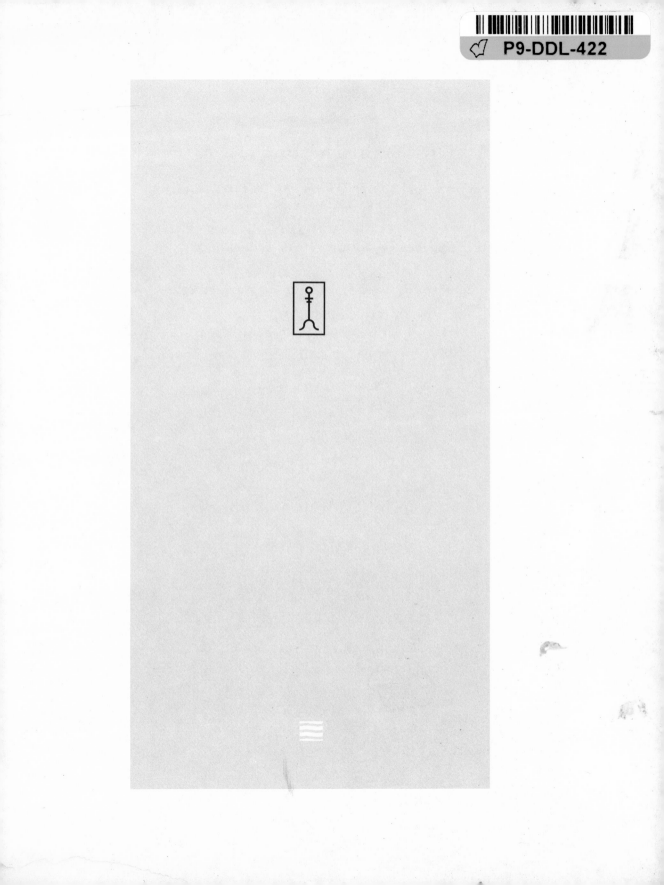

## Also by Sarah, The Duchess of York

*Reinventing Yourself with The Duchess of York:*
*Inspiring Stories and Strategies*

*Win the Weight Game:*
*Successful Strategies for Living Well*

*Dieting with The Duchess:*
*Secrets and Sensible Advice for a Great Body*

*Dining with The Duchess:*
*Making Everyday Meals a Special Occasion*

*The Palace of Westminster*

*Victoria and Albert:*
*Life at Osborne House*

*Travels with Queen Victoria*

*My Story*


## Also by Weight Watchers

*Great Cooking Every Day*

*The Fit Factor*

*Simply the Best Italian*

*New Complete Cookbook*

*Stop Stuffing Yourself:*
*7 Steps to Conquering Overeating*

*Simply the Best:*
*250 Prizewinning Family Recipes*

*. . . and many more*

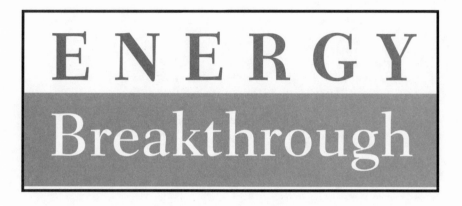

# ENERGY Breakthrough

## JUMP-START YOUR WEIGHT LOSS AND FEEL GREAT

## Sarah,
### The Duchess of York
### *and* Weight Watchers

A FIRESIDE BOOK
PUBLISHED BY SIMON & SCHUSTER
NEW YORK  LONDON  TORONTO
SYDNEY  SINGAPORE

FIRESIDE
Rockefeller Center
1230 Avenue of the Americas
New York, NY 10020

First Fireside Edition 2003

FIRESIDE and colophon are registered trademarks of Simon & Schuster, Inc.

Weight Watchers is a registered trademark of Weight Watchers International, Inc.

For information about special discounts for bulk purchases, please contact
Simon & Schuster Special Sales: 1-800-456-6798 or business@simonandschuster.com

DESIGNED BY DEBORAH KERNER/DANCING BEARS DESIGN
Manufactured in the United States of America
10   9   8   7   6   5   4   3   2   1
Library of Congress Cataloging-in-Publication data is available.

ISBN 0-7432-2620-8
    0-7432-3286-0 (Pbk)

A WORD ABOUT WEIGHT WATCHERS

Since 1963, Weight Watchers has grown from a handful of people to millions of members annually. Today, Weight Watchers is recognized as one of the leading names in safe and sensible weight control. Weight Watchers members form a diverse group, from youths to senior citizens, attending meetings around the globe.

Although weight-loss and weight-management results vary by individual, we recommend that you attend Weight Watchers meetings, follow the Weight Watchers food plan, and participate in regular physical activity. For the Weight Watchers meeting nearest you, call 1-800-651-6000. Visit our Web site at WeightWatchers.com

Weight Watchers Publishing Group        Creative and Editorial Director: Nancy Gagliardi
Publishing Assistant: Jenny Laboy-Brace        Text: Stacey Colino, M.S.        Food Editor: Eileen Runyan
Recipe Developers: Maureen Luchejko, Eileen Runyan
Photography: Ann Stratton        Food Stylist: Rori Trovato        Prop Stylist: Cathy Cook
Editorial and art produced by W/W Twentyfirst Corp., 360 Lexington Ave., New York, NY 10017

PHOTO CREDITS: Following page 32: First page: (top) Louise Dyer; (bottom) Constantino Ruspoli. Second page: (top) Constantino Ruspoli; (bottom left and right) courtesy of Weight Watchers International. Third page: (top left) Louise Dyer; (top right, bottom left) personal archive. Fourth page: Constantino Ruspoli. All other photographs by Ann Stratton.

# Contents

≡

≡

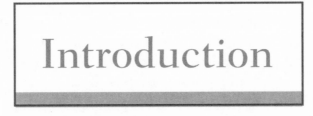

# Introduction

BY SARAH, THE DUCHESS OF YORK

Everywhere I go these days people ask me where I get the energy to do all the things I do. It's a good question, and sometimes I don't know the answer myself. Yet the one thing I do know is that I just keep going forward rather than trying to resist my momentum. You see, I am grateful for my life today and I'd not be where I am had I not learned to harness my energy and take the kinds of risks you need to take in order to get what you want. Writing my last book for Weight Watchers, *Reinventing Yourself,* made me realize just how far I'd come.

Since I have two teens at home, a busy career in America, and charity work that takes me all over the globe, you can bet there are times when I feel utterly exhausted. I can also tell you, though, that I've never felt more energized. This book is designed to help you rediscover and revitalize your energy level, first with an assessment of your life and lifestyle to pinpoint where your energy comes from, and second, by identifying ways in which your energy can be sapped. In my experience, nothing drains away energy quite like stress: You know you are overwhelmed, but don't know what to do about it. Like many women, I'm a multitasker and juggler who can simultaneously think, walk, and talk, all the while balancing a teacup standing on one foot. The sheer volume of tasks I juggle today is greater than ever, but instead of feeling bedraggled as I used to, now my energy reserve stays high.

What has changed?

Through a healthy diet, exercise, and a positive attitude, I've learned how to keep my engine in top condition. Reassessing my priorities and planning my life around them has made a tremendous difference, too.

In the days following my separation from Andrew, I could do little more than lie in bed with the curtains drawn. My life was in shambles, and the chaos and negativity surrounding me made it impossible to think clearly about how to pick up the pieces. The profound sorrow and shame I felt over the loss of my marriage left me reeling emotionally. And I was physically depleted, an ironic state for the woman everyone had dubbed as "fun, feisty Fergie," and a "breath of fresh air." It had taken years for me to reach the depths, and I am the first to admit that it was largely my own insecurities and unhealthy lifestyle that led to my fall.

I could not have been more in love when I married in 1986, and back then I had boundless energy as I embarked on my new life as the Duchess of York. In time, however, the stress of public life and my desire to please everybody became almost unbearable. The constant scrutiny and nonstop criticism fed my innate insecurity to the point that I felt unsuitable as a wife and mother. In essence, I felt like an absolute failure. My problem with weight was a clear indication that I was terribly unhappy, and looking back I can see why my countless quick-fix diets were like desperate gasps for air. In the end, the dreary cloud of negativity that permeated my life brought my world crashing down. Had it not been for my girls, Beatrice and Eugenie, I wonder how I'd ever have managed to get back up on my feet again.

For me, an important first step was becoming physically active again. Just the routine of a simple workout gave me a reason to get up in the morning. I started to eat better and that gave me energy too, but I still struggled with the impulse to binge whenever something upset me. There was genuinely plenty to worry about, not the least of which was how I would go about supporting myself as a single mother. My divorce settlement was small and I still faced paying back a huge bank overdraft, so when Weight Watchers approached me in 1996 to be its U.S. spokesperson, I was eager to work. However, despite my good fortune, the anxiety I felt over this new chapter of my life was overwhelming, and I admit the anxiety robbed me of the enthusiasm I should have felt.

I remember feeling numb when I walked onstage at the Weight Watchers press conference to announce my new role as spokesperson. The ballroom at the Pierre Hotel in New York City was jam-packed with press—literally spread wall to wall with reporters, editors, photographers, and TV cameras. I'd come to fear the press back home, but somehow I mustered enough nerve to get on with the program and deliver my speech. In photos from that day I can see that my hair and makeup were overdone compared to my natural look now; even my clothes seemed to be serving as camouflage.

In England, news of my new job was not well received, and it spawned an outpouring of negativity about my pursuit of a paying career. If you can imagine the glares and stares that awaited me as I came through London's Heathrow Airport, you can understand how the renewed criticism of my commercial life and actions successfully squelched any optimism I'd felt about my new career. I was fighting for my future and for some dignity. I think it was adrenaline and my survivor instinct that convinced me to ignore the critics and just get on with it all.

My responsibility to Weight Watchers was reason enough to get on track with a healthy eating and fitness regimen. People who know me know that I am a person of absolute integrity; I speak from the heart, so I couldn't possibly take on the job of promoting the diet without actually doing it myself. It's said that the truth will set you free, and coming to America to speak openly about my personal battle with weight had a profoundly cathartic effect on me. From the start, I hit the road making personal appearances at Weight Watchers meetings. I crisscrossed the country. The trips were physically demanding and emotionally exhausting, with reporters questioning me at every turn about very personal parts of my life. But this sort of forced introspection caused me to start connecting the dots of my past, and in doing so, I found myself gaining fresh insight about who I was, where my life had taken me, and where I wanted to go. I was shaky and unsure of myself, hardly an icon for health or success. But somehow I managed to assume my new role thanks mostly to the enormous outpouring of support and goodwill that I received from thousands of Weight Watchers members who didn't come out to judge me as a fallen royal, but rather to cheer me on as one of their own.

I spend a great deal of time in America these days, and I really enjoy it. In fact, I take every opportunity to thank Americans from the bottom of my heart because, with their encouragement, I've had the faith and energy to move on in my life.

So that's my story. Now I want to know, what is yours? Do you find yourself always tired, just barely dragging yourself through the day? Or are you facing a particularly rough road ahead and want to ensure that your stamina will stay high?

We all live in the age of stress. I think women face a particularly demanding kind of stress because we wear so many hats. Unlike our mother's generation, we are more in touch with our own needs and aspirations, which, paradoxically, can be both liberating and stressful. If you are feeling overwhelmed in your life, chances are that you feel lacking in energy and drained of vitality.

The problem is, how do you stop that lack of energy cycle? It's probably all you can do to stay where you are right now. But here's a fact: there's no single step to break this cycle. You will have to evaluate your general state of health and your diet and exercise habits; you'll also need to honestly assess trouble areas that weigh heavily on your mind. If how you live now leaves you drained of energy, accept that something in your life may have to change. Only you can put a realistic plan into action and I urge you to find the courage to want to make a change in your life. Yes, that step into the unknown is frightening, but what have you got to lose if holding back will keep you feeling tired, saddened, and unhappy in your own skin?

In the coming chapters, we'll cover various ways that nutrition, exercise, and attitude can help give you energy. But I want you to keep in mind that the best diet and greatest trainers in the world won't work unless you can energize your soul, too. When your mind, body, and soul are energized, you'll feel as though nothing can ever hold you back.

# PART 1

# Understanding Energy

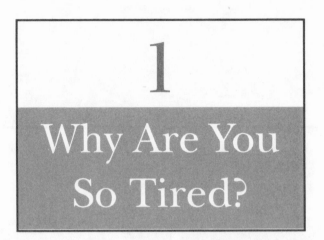

# 1
# Why Are You So Tired?

**D**rop a stone in a pool of water, and the ripples will spread in all directions. It's amazing how that bit of energy in one spot soon affects a much larger area. I see my charity work in much the same way: a nucleus of positive and focused energy that elicits waves of more positive energy, spreading itself out to the point where something unimaginably big is accomplished. The same can be said for how a positive attitude and a healthy lifestyle work together in ways that make us feel energized and alive.

Many things in my life give me energy. Once I started paying attention to what I was eating and how certain foods made me feel, I became a firm believer in the power of good nutrition. Certainly eating the right, healthy foods is like putting high-octane gas in my tank. Just as I know I will feel pumped up on days when I'm eating well, I also now know that skipping meals or filling up on empty calories will sap my energy. The same thing holds true for my exercise routine: sticking to my morning workout not only gets my body revved up, it boosts my mood, too. In fact, I physically miss the good feeling I have when I'm active, which is why I try to fit in even a short version of my workout when traveling takes me away from my normal routine.

I recall years ago when I had the experience of a lifetime trekking in the Himalayas of Nepal, certainly one of the most rugged and spectacularly beautiful places I'd ever seen. Our Sherpa guides, native to this remote region of the world, are renowned for their mountaineering skill as well as for their incredible stamina, and I learned a great deal from them about setting goals and using strategy to achieve them. Mountain trekking can be physically and emotionally grueling, and the extreme conditions can make you acutely aware of how your mind and body work together to give you energy. I recall staring up at the peak we were about to ascend, wondering where on earth I'd find the energy to trek ten thousand feet up to our final destination. Of course it takes days to complete such a trip, and the prospect of doing it would have been a lot less daunting in my mind had I just broken it down into smaller, more manageable parts. That trip taught me what it means to take one day at a time. Some of the obstacles I faced early on made me feel like turning back, partly because my normal haste and picky eating habits did not work up in the mountains. The thin air could have sapped all of my energy, so I had no choice but to pace myself and eat what I was given. Each day was a new milestone for me, and my confidence soared as we progressed until we finally reached base camp. My body literally took me to astounding new heights, and I can tell you that the lessons I learned at the top of the world apply just as well back in London.

Travel plays a critical role in my life. Sometimes I'm on the road so much that I feel as if I lead two separate lives: one Sarah lives in England, while the other Sarah lives wherever her career happens to take her. I have had to learn to adapt my diet and fitness routines for both Sarahs, and it's my ability to be flexible with what I do that assures me that I'll always have the energy reserve I need.

When I'm at home in Britain, my first priority is being a great mother to Beatrice and Eugenie, who still attend day school near our home outside London. Most mornings are quite ordinary: we sit down to breakfast at 7:30 A.M., then I catch fifteen minutes of television news as I get myself together before I'm off to drop Beatrice and Eugenie at school. Then it's back home to start my day.

Since I don't do commercial work in Britain, I spend much of my time helping run Children in Crisis and Chances for Children, the two charities I founded while also serving as patron to organizations such as Tommy's Fund, the Teenage Cancer Trust, and Interplast. With encouragement from UNICEF, I am now directing con-

## 5 THINGS I KNOW ABOUT ENERGY

1. Energy is the key to a life full of joy and vitality.

2. Energy is my reward for eating well, exercising, resting, and having a positive attitude.

3. Energy is drained by negativity.

4. Energy opens doors and, at times, even carries me through difficult times.

5. Energy is contagious.

siderable energy to supporting the plight of children in Africa who are stigmatized or ostracized by their tribe because their parents are suffering from HIV or have died of AIDS.

Yet my work in Britain takes me all over Europe. It's a rare day that I sit down at a desk and simply work. Being on the run can make it hard to eat nutritiously, and the stress of running from one appointment to the next can be wearing. To keep my life from becoming a complete circus, I structure my workdays in ways that provide for balance and efficiency. After I drop the girls off at school, I have my workout with my trainer, Josh. I've become quite protective of my workout time with him, because for me, being healthy and fit is an investment in myself today and in my future. Usually I hop onto my exercise bike and ride. It really gets my heart pumping, plus I can get a jump on my day. My time on the exercise bike is perfect for catching up on the news.

Through the rest of my day, I try to use my time wisely. Shuttling between appointments, I check lists, read my mail, and make business calls. I also schedule meetings in the late morning and midafternoon so I can be home when Beatrice and Eugenie return from school. Sitting down to tea with the girls each afternoon not only maintains our special bond but enables me to stay aware of what's happening in their lives (so important in this day and age). Our downtime together, I've discovered, is also a way for me to slow down and regroup—which produces more energy. I still enjoy going out some evenings and look forward to seeing friends, but there are many nights when I am just as happy to stay in and simply go to bed early.

One more thought: even though I may be terribly busy at home, I always try to do a bit of the things I love. When I can, I still manage to write my children's stories, paint landscapes, and shoot photographs. These creative outlets are exciting and, ultimately, energizing. In other words, positive fun begets positive energy.

## Get Support

Being surrounded by positive, like-minded people can be thoroughly energizing. I experience this positive energy at Weight Watchers "Super Meetings," huge gatherings sometimes in excess of a thousand members, who come out to hear me speak about my issue with weight, and where we all share in applauding the success of fellow members. You can't help but feel charged up after one of these events, and I can't think of a better example of the powers of group support and positive thinking.

# Curse of the Superwoman

More responsibilities, less free time. More stress, less sleep. More daily hassles, less serenity in your life. Call it the curse of the contemporary Superwoman. If you're like many women, you probably try to pack as much into your days and nights as possible. You manage to muster enough time and energy to put together the family lunches, organize the car pool, take the pet to the vet, put in a full day's work, check in with an ailing friend or relative, listen to your spouse vent about his day, prepare dinner, help with homework and baths, and tidy up the house at the end of the day. Doing it all might even be a point of pride—a sign of a full, successful life or evidence of your competence and ability to juggle multiple commitments. And it is all of that which should make you feel incredibly good about what you're accomplishing.

Between having a career, raising kids, tending to your family, keeping up with your friends, taking care of your household, and fulfilling all the other tasks of modern life, you're pulling off an amazing feat. But the important—yet often overlooked—question is, at what price? The truth is, many modern women are absolutely exhausted, physically, emotionally, and spiritually. Their batteries are sorely in need of recharging. Many feel as though they are the walking wounded. And many are flirting with an energy crisis that could rival the gas shortage of the 1970s.

These days, energy probably seems like an incredibly precious commodity that's climbing up your endangered resources list, precisely because it's in such short supply. For instance, day after day, you might find yourself continuously hitting the snooze button on your alarm and dragging yourself out of bed. You might have trouble thinking clearly or concentrating during the day, or you might pump yourself with coffee all day just to keep going, or you might wind up on the verge of tears by 5 P.M. simply because you're so drained. Come 9 P.M.? You might feel as though you could become the next Rip Van Winkle and sleep for twenty years.

Why is that? Probably because the more you take on, the more your lifestyle could wind up dragging you down: when too-much-to-do-in-too-little-time becomes a way of life and you start to feel pulled in as many directions as Gumby, you're in danger of having your stress level soar and your energy vanish into a black hole. Indeed, for many women, the only private time they have is in the shower—and even that may be interrupted by a kid with a crisis. During the day, you may be so busy running from home to work to errands and back again that you barely have time to catch your breath. Or collect your thoughts. Or do something—anything—nice for yourself.

No wonder research has found that the incidence of fatigue is higher among women than men. It's also one of the primary reasons women consult their doctors. In a 1998 study at the University of Toronto, researchers sought to examine the major health concerns of 153 women, and not surprisingly, fatigue ranked at the top of the list among nearly a third and among the top ten concerns among 80 percent of the women. To what exactly did the women attribute their fatigue? Interestingly enough, they were more likely to blame social and personal factors than their health. In descending order of importance, they ascribed their fatigue to the following culprits:

- Working both inside and outside the home
- Poor sleep
- Lack of time for themselves
- Lack of exercise
- Financial worries
- Relationship troubles
- Emotional factors
- Taking care of ill family members
- A scarcity of social and personal support
- Poor physical health

Meanwhile, in a study of women's beliefs regarding persistent fatigue at the University of Missouri–Columbia, the researcher concluded that "long-term fatigue is ubiquitous in the lives of many women and . . . many perceive role burden and stress to be important contributing factors."

## THE MISSING (GENETIC) LINK

We all know women who seem to have limitless amounts of energy, who can be on the run from dawn till dusk—and still manage to have flawlessly manicured nails, perfectly well-behaved kids, and an impeccably neat house. Meanwhile, we're barely dragging ourselves through the day. What accounts for these differences?

To a certain extent, your energy level may be inherited, although researchers haven't uncovered the full story as far as genetic influences go. But studies with twins, for example, have suggested that hyperactivity is partly inherited. Research has also found that people with manic personalities are usually born that way. What's more, an individual's metabolism can be inherited from her parents—and it may be that energy levels are similarly passed down from one generation to the next.

But your energy level can also be a product of nature and nurture—a result of the interplay between biology, your lifestyle habits, your personality and outlook, and the events in your life. So while researchers continue to tease out the genetic influences on energy, you can begin to address the other factors that can have a big impact on your get up and go.

## How Did I Get So Tired?

While you might chalk up an energy deficit as the inevitable result of lack of sleep, too much work, or getting older, it's your complicated lifestyle that's more likely to blame—a serious concern when you consider that persistent exhaustion can seriously compromise the quality of your days, as well as your physical and emotional well-being. After all, when you feel as though you're constantly running on empty, how much enjoyment or pleasure can you actually derive from what you're doing? How can you fully experience the moments of your life, and how can you tend to your own physical and emotional needs when you barely have enough time to take care of everyone else?

On the most basic level, when you're already feeling dead tired, it's hard to muster the energy to eat right and exercise regularly or to try to lose weight. Here's a reality check: carrying around extra pounds can actually sap your energy, which can set you up for a vicious circle. Because you might lack the motivation to make healthy changes to your life or your weight, you simply maintain the sluggish status quo. You might wind up eating even more than usual in an effort to boost your energy, which could lead to further weight gain if you don't burn off the extra calories. Or you may vegetate on the couch because you can't summon the strength to go for a walk or a jog. The trouble is, sticking with poor eating habits and a sedentary lifestyle—regardless of your weight—can leave you feeling depleted of energy.

Yet consider the results if you actually did something about it: For example, a study at Austin Peay State University in Clarksville, Tennessee, found that when overweight women lost weight, the severity of their fatigue declined along with the number on the scale. Moreover, there are several correlations between fatigue and excess weight, according to medical experts. On an intuitive level, carrying excess weight can be very tiring for the body, but other factors may come into play as well, including depression, stress, and poor exercise and eating habits. Depression or a constant state of stress could be fueling an emotional eating habit. And being out of shape—in poor physical condition, in other words—can also make you feel tired. But there also may be a chemical component at work. In a study at the Sleep Research and Treatment Center at the Pennsylvania State University College of Medicine, researchers found that daytime sleepiness was much more common among obese people; they concluded that it may be due to a metabolic and/or circadian abnormality that afflicts those who are overweight. One thing is certain: if you're low on energy and overweight, shedding pounds will help you regain the bounce in your step.

Indeed, when it comes to both energy and weight control, doing something—whether being physically activite or following a healthy diet—is better than doing nothing. A recent study from Kuwait University found that even if physical activity isn't frequent enough for aerobic conditioning, it can lead to a lower body fat content than if a person is completely inactive. Meanwhile, a study from the University of Colorado Health Sciences Center in Denver examined the effects of occasional physical inactivity on a high-fat or high-carbohydrate diet. The findings: consistently consuming a high-carbohydrate diet could provide some protection against the accumulation of body fat in those who have a pattern of exercise that includes frequent sedentary days; the same cannot be said for those who consume a high-fat diet. With either lifestyle change, you'd likely experience a renewed lightness of being and a boost in your energy.

# Understanding the Energy Equation

Fatigue is a subjective state, and what sparks it for one woman may be quite different from what triggers it for another. A person's responses to life events are so individual, and research has found, again and again, that it's a person's perception or reaction to a situation that determines whether it's stressful, exhausting, or invigorating. Indeed, the concept of energy has more to do with feeling than with physiology. A multitude of variables come together and affect what you feel as energy—or lack thereof—and the psychological variables can quickly override the physical factors. Whatever the underlying causes may be, fatigue is sometimes defined, in the world of medicine, as "a sustained sense of exhaustion with reduced motivation and capacity for physical and/or mental activity."

While it's true that many serious illnesses number fatigue among their primary symptoms, for the vast majority of women, fatigue is a sign of an energy drain—and nothing more. It's an SOS that your energy balance is out of whack, a wake-up call that something is amiss with the way you're running your life. In a sense, fatigue is a positive thing because it is sending you essential information about the state of your affairs. It's telling you to reevaluate your life and find ways to boost your energy so that you can improve the quality of your life.

Think of the energy equation as an old-fashioned scale (like the scales of justice, not the type you weigh yourself on): In order for your energy to be in a state of balance, the amount of energy you expend through exercise, mental strain, work, stress, and so on must be replenished by the energy you conserve or reserve with smart eating habits, physical fitness, pleasure, and other positive factors. When the energy you're expending is adequately replenished with good self-care, your energy scales are well balanced—and you'll likely feel a sense of vim and vigor.

You probably already know that good eating and sleep habits can increase your energy level. But you may not realize that the energy deficit you may be experiencing is probably the result not only of the stress and added responsibility but also of the pleasure and relaxation that's disappeared. Because there are so many different forms of personal energy—physical, emotional, spiritual, sensual, and so on—igniting your vitality requires far more than simply eating nutritious food. Many other activities can jump-start your sense of vitality. You might feel absolutely invigorated after playing a raucously fun game of tag with your kids or after going for a walk and getting fresh air on a sunny day. You might feel as though your batteries recharged after getting a night of deep, uninterrupted sleep or after talking with a close friend who makes you laugh. You might feel inspired after working hard on a project you feel passionately about or engaging in a hobby like painting or gardening that brings you boundless pleasure. All of this is the good stuff of life—and of energy.

When it comes right down to it, the energy equation is all about synergy: your eating and exercise habits, your scheduling practices, the level of rest and relaxation in your life, the pleasure you allow yourself, and even your weight can have a dynamic effect on each other. Having optimal energy is a matter of achieving the right balance: eat enough food but not too much; consume nutritionally rich foods, rather than empty calories; treat your body to regular movement and your mind to plenty of high-quality time that's just for you—and you'll create lots of high-octane energy. What's more, this can help you get on your way to healthy weight management and good health. In this state, many aspects of your life will probably begin to feel more manageable, more possible, more promising. Suddenly, your life may no longer feel as out of control as it once did. And feeling is believing.

In fact, studies have found that self-efficacy—a can-do spirit or a sense that you have the will and the way to accomplish your goals—can be pivotal in making lifestyle changes. In one study of normal and overweight adults, researchers at Baylor College of Medicine in Houston found that people whose weight didn't fluctuate over a one-year period had a significantly higher sense of well-being, greater self-efficacy when it came to eating behaviors, and lower stress than those whose weight changed. More recently, a study at Miriam Hospital and Brown University School of Medicine in Providence, Rhode Island, found that overweight women who shed pounds in a twelve-week weight-management program experienced significant improvements in self-efficacy when it came to eating, exercise, and other health habits.

This kind of thing doesn't amount to a miraculous transformation. Generally speaking, energy—as well as a sense of general well-being—is something you either fuel or fizzle by the choices you make on a daily basis. Which is good news because this means that you have the power to reclaim your lost energy—or to boost what you already have. But it also means that the responsibility for improving your energy quotient lies solely with you. So you may have to get off the constantly revolving carousel of life for a bit and think about what you want and what you're currently doing with your actions. You may need to make a conscious decision to stop running on adrenaline (or toxic fumes) or being driven by fear. You may need to set new priorities in order to make it possible to carve out time to prepare healthy meals, exercise consistently, and devote time to spiritual renewal. In other words, you may need to put yourself back on your own radar screen and begin to cater to your personal energy needs.

## ARE YOU SICK AND TIRED?

Myriad health conditions include fatigue among their primary symptoms. But more often than not, these conditions cause other physical symptoms, too, so try to become aware of any additional changes in how you feel. If you notice any of the other symptoms that could point to one of the following conditions, it's time to schedule a doctor's appointment. Even if you don't, you'd be smart to consult your doctor since many low-grade infections (such as mononucleosis, sinusitis, and Lyme disease) and other medical conditions (such as heart disease) can also cause long-lasting fatigue.

**ALLERGIES:** When your immune system reacts inappropriately or overly intensely to substances such as plants, foods, animal dander, chemicals, or even medicines, you may experience a battery of symptoms. Depending on the offending culprit, these can include an itchy nose and throat, sneezing, coughing, watery eyes, skin rashes, digestive distress—and, of course, a drop in energy from this physiological overreaction. Pinpointing the problematic agent isn't always easy, but your doctor can help with this as well as with treating your symptoms.

**ANEMIA:** Whether it stems from an iron deficiency or another underlying cause, this is a condition in which the concentration of the oxygen-carrying pigment in the blood—hemoglobin—is below normal. As a result, you may experience headaches, dizziness, lethargy, and tiredness, among other symptoms. A simple blood test can diagnose anemia.

**DEPRESSION:** Feeling tired or low on energy is one of the warning signs of depression, but it's often accompanied by feelings of sadness, hopelessness, moodiness, pessimism, sleep and appetite disturbances, and/or a general loss of interest in activities that used to be pleasurable. It's widely estimated that one in four women will suffer major depression at some point in her life. So if any of these symptoms describes you, it may be time to seek professional help.

**DIABETES:** In this metabolic disorder, the body is unable to produce or respond properly to the hormone insulin. As a result, frequent urination and thirst, unexplained fatigue, hunger, weakness, or vision problems can result. But it's often a silent disorder: approximately 16 million people in the United States have diabetes, according to the American Diabetes Association, but nearly a third of them don't even know it. If you have any of these symptoms, have your blood sugar tested without delay.

**FIBROMYALGIA:** Though pain, particularly in the muscles and tendons, usually accompanies this condition, fatigue is also a prominent symptom of fibromyalgia, a connective tissue disorder that's a close cousin to arthritis. By some estimates, women of childbearing age make up 80 percent of patients with fibromyalgia. Generally, a doctor will diagnose the condition by testing for trigger points for pain along various muscles.

**SLEEP PROBLEMS:** Sleep apnea—a disorder in which someone stops breathing for ten seconds or longer during sleep—and other forms of sleep-disordered breathing, including snoring, are more common among people who are overweight. The reason: in those who are carrying extra pounds, the upper airway is encroached upon by the fat pads on either side of the airway, which can make it susceptible to collapsing during sleep. This makes breathing more difficult—and causes tiredness during the day. Surgery and other medical treatments can often correct the problem, but losing weight can also improve sleep-disordered breathing problems considerably.

**THYROID DISORDERS:** When the thyroid gland becomes underactive, a condition called hypothyroidism, you may experience weight gain, lethargy, dry skin, hair loss, cold intolerance, constipation, and other unpleasant symptoms. Women are especially prone to this condition as they get older. Fortunately, a special blood test can detect the condition, and medication can treat it effectively.

## MEDICATIONS AND ENERGY: A POTENT COCKTAIL

It's no secret that many medications can cause drowsiness and fatigue. But sometimes the effects are subtle enough that you may not realize that a drug you're taking could be sapping your energy or interfering with your sleep, leading to fatigue the next day. If you suspect that a medication may be causing your exhaustion, talk to your doctor. Individual reactions to specific drugs are so varied that even if sleepiness or fatigue isn't a common side effect, it doesn't necessarily mean a drug isn't affecting you in that way. Here are several commonly taken medications that can compromise your energy:

Antianxiety drugs

Antibiotics

Antidepressants

Antihistamines

Antispasmodic drugs

Asthma medications

Cold remedies

High-blood-pressure medications

Painkillers

## The Natural Rhythms of Energy

The truth is, many people expect energy to be a constant in their lives and they're disappointed when it's not. We've become such a twenty-four-hour society—with our cell phones, home computers, fax machines and beepers—that the boundaries dividing home, work, and family have blurred. These days, we never truly leave work behind; it follows us wherever we go, and, as a result, we may feel as though we're on call all the time. Indeed, a recent study by the Families and Work Institute in New York City found that nearly one-third of employees in the United States often or very often feel overworked or overwhelmed by the amount of work they have to do. Not surprisingly, the institute's 1997 National Study of the Changing Workforce found that employees with highly demanding jobs and not-so-supportive workplaces experience more stress, worse moods, and less energy when they're away from their jobs—"all of which jeopardize their personal and family well-being," according to the report.

Part of the problem is that the pressure to continuously perform at your peak has increased so much that there is little tolerance for any variation. But this expectation is unrealistic because your personal energy naturally ebbs and flows in cycles throughout the day, week, month, and seasons. Upon awakening in the morning, your energy level usually rises as your body temperature does, peaking just before noon. Research has found that many people say they are most alert and their reasoning skills are high at 11 A.M.; meanwhile, the ability to make complex decisions peaks around noon. A person's energy generally slumps after lunch, sometime between 2 and 4 P.M., before rising again slightly until early evening. From there, it gradually goes down until about 9 P.M., when most people begin to slip into a somewhat soporific state. Of course, these shifts may vary if you're a lark (a morning person) or an owl (you feel your best at night), but the general pattern is likely to be similar.

If you typically feel more energetic over the weekend, that's not due to biology: you're probably getting a little more sleep and experiencing less stress than during the week, which can put the spring back in your step. But it could also be your state of mind. If you're stuck in a ho-hum job that bores you or you don't get along with your boss, lifting that burden may be enough to jump-start your energy when you're at home. As welcome as that weekend energy boost may be, it's telling you something about how or where you're spending your week.

## YOUR ENERGY JOURNAL

Before you can give yourself an energy makeover, you'll need to discover your own natural peaks and valleys as well as the lifestyle and mood factors that influence them. The best way to do this is to monitor your energy levels and habits throughout the day for a week, ideally midway through the menstrual cycle (not when you have PMS!), then to look for potential links between your energy level and certain situations. Once you've done this, you'll be in a better position to take steps to improve your energy quotient.

How to start? Take a notebook or a legal pad and at the top of each page note the date, how much sleep you got the previous night, and what the quality of your sleep was. Then, mark four columns horizontally: time, energy/mood quotient (rated from one to five, with one being low and five being high), eating/drinking, and activity/situation. Under the time column, write down every hour, from awakening until you typically go to bed, vertically down the page. At the bottom of the page, leave some room for you to jot down "Possible connections" between what's happening in your daily life and your energy level and "Goals" for what you might do differently.

Here's a glimpse of what a sample energy journal might look like:

## SAMPLE ENERGY JOURNAL

DATE: *Monday, January 7*   PREVIOUS NIGHT'S SLEEP: *11 p.m.-7 a.m.*
QUALITY: *So-so. Woke up twice, had trouble falling back to sleep*

| Time | Energy/mood quotient | Eating/drinking | Activity/situation |
|---|---|---|---|
| 7 A.M. | 1=Very sleepy, cranky | 0 | Showered, dressed self and kids, packed lunches |
| 8 A.M. | 2=Less sleepy | Coffee, banana | Got ready for work, dropped kids at school, stopped at dry cleaners |
| 9 A.M. | 3=Alert, cheerful | More coffee | Prepared for meeting, scheduled doctor's appt. and home repairs . . . |
| 12 P.M. | 4=Peppy but wired | Sip of water | Wrote memo |
| 1 P.M. | 2½=Dragging, irritable | Double-cheese pizza at desk, diet soda . . . | Finished memo, called Mother |
| 3 P.M. | 1½=Nearly comatose | Coffee | Yawned through meeting and so on until . . . |
| 10 P.M. | 1=Wiped out | Herb tea | Planned schedule for tomorrow, tidied house, read over presentation before lights out |

**Possible connections:** Didn't sleep well; relied on lots of coffee to stay alert; ate high-calorie lunch for energy but felt slump anyway; stuck inside for long hours

**Goals:** Try to take a walk outside and squeeze in exercise to boost energy and alertness.

While social reasons may make women more susceptible to periodic energy drains than men are, physical attributes may also play a role. As Holly Atkinson, M.D., author of *Women and Fatigue,* notes, "Women have smaller bodies with less muscle mass than men, leading them to suffer from physical exhaustion sooner than the average male." Plus, fatigue is a hallmark of many of the milestones in a woman's reproductive life (puberty, menstruation, pregnancy, and menopause), which are associated with fluctuations in estrogen and progesterone. But there is quite a bit of individuality here, too. Studies have found that some women experience a burst of energy, creativity, and awareness just before they get their period each month. Other women, especially those prone to premenstrual syndrome (PMS), feel sluggish and sore before the start of their periods. In addition, many women report greater feelings of well-being and self-esteem right after ovulation, when estrogen levels peak.

Meanwhile, people who live in northern climates often have lower energy during the winter months. In a study involving more than six hundred adults, researchers at the University of Massachusetts found that feelings of depression, hostility, anger, irritability, and anxiety were highest in the winter and lowest in the summer. They noted that exposure to light, as well as diet and activity levels, varies with the seasons, which could explain these mood differences that can act as a drain upon your physical and emotional energy. Spring and fall, by contrast, tend to bring a renewed sense of vitality to many people.

## The Epidemic of Exhaustion

In these hard-driving times, many people fight their natural energy peaks and valleys and expect themselves to exhibit optimal performance seven days a week, fifty-two weeks a year. But it's just not possible to operate with the same level of intensity and vitality all the time. What we need to do, instead, is learn to honor our natural energy rhythms instead of working against them. When your physical and emotional stamina is already low, this may require turning down some social invitations so you can make time for much needed rest, setting limits with family members or friends who tend to drain your emotional reserves, or delegating tasks that aren't essential for you to do so that your "to do" list doesn't become insurmountable.

The problem is, when your time and attention are consistently scattered, your energy becomes so diffuse that you wind up wasting much of it. Under such conditions, it's virtually impossible to feel grounded or centered in yourself or mindful of your actions or environment. Besides, when stress becomes a way of life, your body responds by continuously activating its "fight-or-flight" response: the hypothalamus in the brain triggers the release of stress hormones, which in turn influence many different body systems. Being stuck in stress mode consistently depletes the body's energy reserves. It can take a toll on various body systems, causing symptoms such as headaches, insomnia, back pain, diarrhea, weight gain, and frequent colds, among others. And it can have a detrimental effect on your state of mind, robbing you of emotional vim and vigor.

There's no question: when fatigue becomes a fact of everyday life for a healthy adult, your habits, your choices, or your lifestyle are probably to blame. You may feel exhausted simply because being sapped of energy has become the norm for you; it's become the state of your existence. And that's a choice, perhaps a passive one but still a choice because you allowed it to happen. So if you want to rev up your body's engine and recapture the energy you've lost, it's up to you to take charge of doing so. When it comes to the energy equation, there are no quick cures or magic bullets. Contrary to what many advertisers would like you to believe, you can't pop a pill or swallow a potion and suddenly have more vim and vigor than you know what to do with. If you want to jump-start your energy, you're going to have to tinker with your lifestyle.

This doesn't mean you'll necessarily have to give it an overhaul. In all likelihood, you'll be able to continue many of the activities and roles you've embraced; you may just need to alter how you support yourself so that you can better engage in them. The reality is, juggling multiple roles doesn't have to lead to an energy deficit. Several studies have actually found that the more roles a woman has—as a mother, spouse, daughter, worker, friend, and so on—the more physical and psychological well-being she's likely to experience. Of course, it depends on how much she actually enjoys those roles. So if volunteering to help with your daughter's school play or participating in a book club becomes more of an energy buster than an energy booster, you may want to think twice about continuing such commitments.

The key is to set yourself up for energy in all aspects of your life—and you have the power to do this. It involves devising strategic plans for eating and exercising, revamping the lifestyle habits and environmental factors that are pulling the plug on your natural energy resources, and giving yourself an attitude adjustment to promote positive mental energy and eliminate negative energy sappers. Yes, this will require a fair amount of effort on your part. Most of all, it will require consistency in your actions if you want to reap optimal energy benefits. But it's worth it. For one thing, it sure beats the alternative. After all, your personal energy crisis can affect every aspect of your life: your physical well-being, your emotional equilibrium, the quality of your relationships and your social life, even your spiritual outlook.

So when fatigue sets in, take it seriously. Heed its red-alert signal, and try to restore your body's energy balance. You can do this in many different ways but all involve either restoring spent or squandered energy (by consuming nutritious food, drinking lots of water, setting out on a brisk walk, getting some extra shut-eye, breathing deeply, spending time with people who inspire you, and so on) or conserving energy (by taking some quiet time for yourself, passing on nonessential commitments, putting off tasks and chores that don't absolutely have to be done today, or nixing a get-together with a friend who's an energy vampire). Taking these steps will help you elevate your mood and energy.

If you're not sure how to do this on your own, don't worry—that's where Energy Breakthrough comes in. It's not a substitute for a doctor's care if you're suffering an energy deficit as well as symptoms that could signal a medical condition. But it can help you take an unvarnished look at your lifestyle and identify the covert factors that could be robbing you of energy. Then you'll find out how to restore your lost energy by making vital changes to your eating, exercise, emotional, and spiritual habits. In the process, you'll begin to feel better—and you'll gain the enthusiasm and motivation to lose weight and lead a healthier life. You won't regret it. Time spent on your self is worth the investment. It's revitalizing and rejuvenating—for your body, mind, and soul.

### QUIZ: *What Is Your Exhaustion Telling You?*

It's a mistake to ignore your exhaustion; in all likelihood, your fatigue is trying to tell you something important. To gauge the extent of your energy deficit, read the following statements and then mark them True or False, depending on whether they apply to you.

1. My life feels as though it's spinning out of control—and I'm just along for the ride.
2. I'm almost always tired, even after a good night's sleep.
3. Just getting through the day has become a struggle because I often feel as though I'm running on an empty tank of gas.
4. I don't have the energy to stick with a consistent exercise routine.
5. Most days are so harried that it's all I can do to put dinner on the table, let alone a nutritious one.
6. My sense of humor and optimism seem to have disappeared.

7. I'm often plagued with indecision, and sometimes I have trouble concentrating.

8. I'm often cranky or moody, and I frequently overreact to little annoyances.

9. I'm unhappy with my weight, but I'm too tired to do anything about it.

10. My sex drive has headed south; even the thought of getting intimate is exhausting.

Now count up how many statements you marked "True," then read the corresponding analysis. What your exhaustion is broadcasting loud and clear:

**7–10 points: You're running on an empty energy tank.** You're flirting with burnout— and in serious need of an energy makeover. It's time to make cultivating energy and a sense of well-being top priorities in your life.

**4–6 points: You're riding an energy roller coaster.** Your energy may not be in park all the time, but you're clearly squandering some of your get-up-and-go. Aim to find ways to refuel consistently so that you can fulfill goals in many areas of your life.

**0–2 points: You're stalling in neutral now and then.** You're obviously trying to achieve an energy balance in your life, but some aspects are still off-kilter. Time, then, for some fine-tuning in the energy department.

**0 points: You're keeping yourself energized.** If you are not experiencing any of these problems, you've got your energy under control. Congratulations. Keep up the good work!

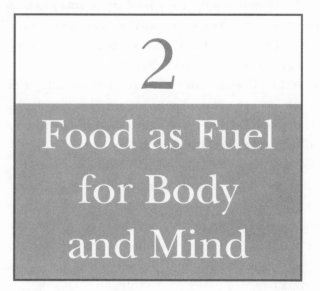

# 2

# Food as Fuel for Body and Mind

At first, coming to work in America was truly frightening to me, and my fear of failure sapped my energy as much as anything I'd faced until then. Out of respect for Her Majesty, I'd decided not to pursue a commercial career in Britain—a decision that meant I'd have to go abroad to earn a living, all while still being a mother to my girls, whose heritage made it necessary for them to grow up in England. Commuting to work across the Atlantic seemed absurd at first, but by staying healthy and fit I've acclimated myself to the long flights and changes in time zones to the point where today I can hop on and off a plane as if it were a city bus.

Yet I'm human, and I do find keeping my energy level high a challenge. My business trips to America can be grueling: often weeks at a time of eighteen-hour days that stretch from before dawn to well after midnight. The demands placed on me while traveling are much different from the stresses I face at home, when I'm living at my normal pace. So I have a much different routine and mind-set on the road; it works well because it takes into account the long days, all the rushing, and quick meals on the fly—all the while making the most of short breaks in between to rest and regroup.

To keep things sane—and my energy up—I try to stay organized. My office gives me updates at intervals during the day rather than calling me at will. I'm getting better at saying "no" to requests, but I still take on too much at times, only to regret it later on. A few years ago when I was on a business trip in the United States, I'd inadvertently agreed to do a live satellite TV interview to Italy at the exact same time as I was to meet with an important group of university scientists. It was quite a dilemma, and I was embarrassed to think that I might have to renege on either commitment, though in the end that wasn't necessary.

But by the end of a busy week, I typically arrive back in England, bleary-eyed but excited to see my girls. Admittedly, I'm always flat out tired and in desperate need of sleep when I get home, but my fatigue now is much different than in the old days, when I was simply overwhelmed by the chaos around me. That chaos or the belief that your life is in chaos is the most exhausting energy drainer there is. Now the satisfaction of having a successful week leaves me uplifted and, crazily enough, thinking about my next trip.

But run out of energy I do. It's what I call "hitting the wall." When I run out of steam, I ask myself why it's happened. Have I taken on too much? Am I getting enough rest? Am I avoiding or worrying about a stressful situation? Have I lapsed on my exercise routine, or maybe I'm not eating as well as I should? Sometimes it's a combination of all these factors, and in the old days being overtired was a sure set up for me to overeat. Through Weight Watchers, I've learned to recognize the symptoms of fatigue and to act to offset them, rather than being weakened by them. For one thing, if I'm feeling hungry *and* exasperated, I try to separate my desire for food from whatever or whoever is making me emotional. It really is far better to deal with

## STAY HYDRATED

"It doesn't have to be a hot day for you to become dehydrated, and the primary symptom is not thirst. If you are dehydrated, you may feel tired, jittery, or have a splitting headache—all clear indications that your body is not functioning properly. Americans have caught on to what Europeans have done for years, which is to carry bottled water when they are out and about."

a problem by picking up the phone rather than a sandwich. And instead of allowing myself to be unreasonably overscheduled, I review my schedule in advance so I can suggest better, realistic ways to get everything done.

I also make my food choices in relation to my energy needs. It's important to find out which foods work best for you. For the life I lead, I've found that I like to consume lean protein, such as chicken breast or plain fish, on days where I need more energy. I love bread, but a breakfast of toast only leaves me hungry a few hours later. For me, an egg-white omelet and some fresh fruit or berries is a much better way to start a busy day. What could be better than a lovely pasta dish at lunch? Some days, nothing. But on days where I need energy to spare, a better choice may be some fish with a smaller side portion of that pasta. I'm also very careful about staying well hydrated, too, drinking enough water to make my daily quota. I love my tea, and indeed a little caffeine boost doesn't hurt. But too much can leave me jittery and very tired, which is why I drink herbal teas in addition to my favorite, Earl Grey.

Learning more about my habits and listening to how my body reacts to them have made me more body- and energy-aware. Now when I sense that I am totally spent and no amount of fitness or healthy eating will turn things right, I take a break. For example, for years I'd heard of a very special spa in Thailand where each day is structured around minding your mind, body, and soul. I finally made the trip last year, and it was a fascinating immersion into Eastern culture, which links physical and emotional harmony with wellness. I arrived quite exhausted, having finished a grueling work schedule in the United States and the end of another hectic school year for my girls. Ten days later I left feeling full of energy and thoroughly rejuvenated, the way a vacation should make you feel. But you don't have to check into a spa to live a balanced life. The tenets of Weight Watchers cover all the bases, giving me the simplicity and structure I rely on every day to lead a balanced life.

# Eating for Energy

Food is the ultimate energy source because it is fuel for your body and mind. Indeed, how, when, and what you eat can have a dramatic effect on your vim and vigor. If you wind up feeling cranky and lethargic by midmorning despite eating breakfast, you may be choosing the wrong foods for the morning meal—likewise, if lunch leaves you in a soporific state or you barely have the energy to drag yourself home at the end of the day. Could it be that your eating habits are squandering your energy resources instead of jump-starting your get-up-and-go? It's possible.

After all, it's important to eat a balanced diet that meets your nutritional needs for the sake of your energy as well as your health. The good news is, you can provide yourself with optimal energy throughout the day if you get smart about eating. It's a matter of fine-tuning the way you choose foods: instead of automatically grabbing whatever is on hand or whatever is easy, you'll need to begin to think about what you eat as part of your own personal energy equation. Consuming nutritious foods at regular intervals throughout the day can help you stay on an even physical and emotional keel by keeping your blood sugar steadier and your energy flowing. But the quality of your food choices counts, as well as the quantity and frequency of your meals. If you want to reap optimal energy, you'll need to say good-bye to careless eating and replace it with a commitment to mindful eating. It's important to understand, however, that what really matters is your individual experience. Based on how your eating habits have affected your energy level in the past, you may want to experiment with different strategies to see what improves your physical and mental vigor.

## DOES DIETING DRAIN YOUR ENERGY?

The answer isn't quite as simple as the question. The reality is that dieting can rob you of energy, but it doesn't have to; the effect depends on how you try to slim down. It's true that low-calorie diets—800 to 1,200 calories per day for women, 800 to 1,400 calories per day for men—as well as very-low-calorie diets, which are defined as less than 800 calories per day, are associated with fatigue. In general, the lower your calorie level drops on a weight-reduction plan, the greater your chances are of feeling tired or listless. In fact, crash diets will simply set your energy up to crash and burn.

But the quality of the calories you consume and the amount of physical activity you get can also influence your energy level. If you were to eat 1,000 calories' worth of glazed doughnuts and be completely sedentary, you would probably ex-

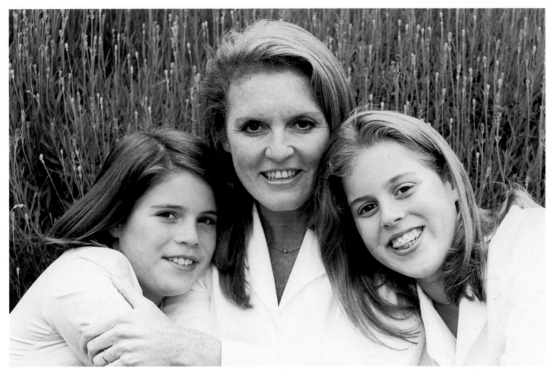

My girls, Beatrice (*left*) and Eugenie (*right*), are the prides of my life. My first and most important job is being their mother, and I schedule my work carefully so I can enjoy what I can of these precious years.

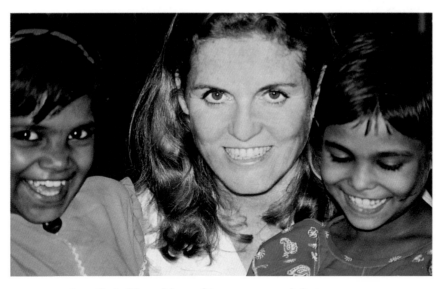

A smile is like a blast of innocence and divine energy.
It can mean so much yet costs nothing at all.

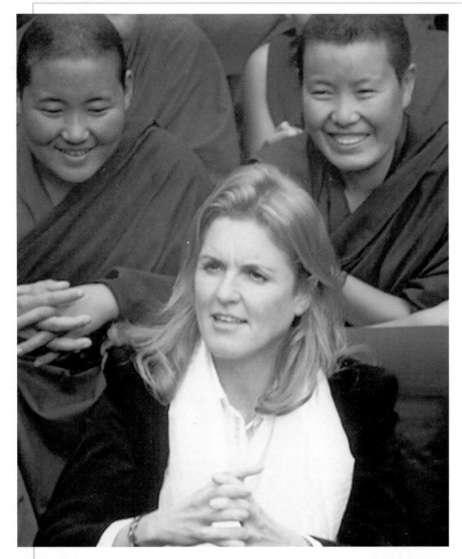

I marvel at the power and serenity of lives guided by dedication, discipline, and unwavering spirit.

(*Below, left*) We all have the capacity to overcome dieting obstacles, which is clear by the amazing weight-loss success stories we share at Weight Watchers meetings.

(*Below, right*) I still get nervous before taking the stage at one of our Weight Watchers Super Meetings, which always draw the press and a huge and enthusiastic crowd.

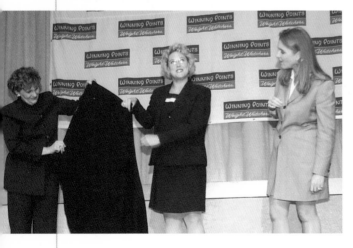

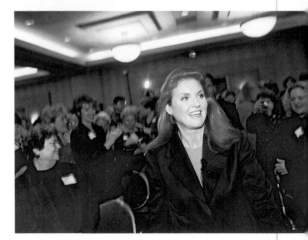

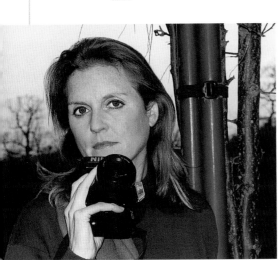

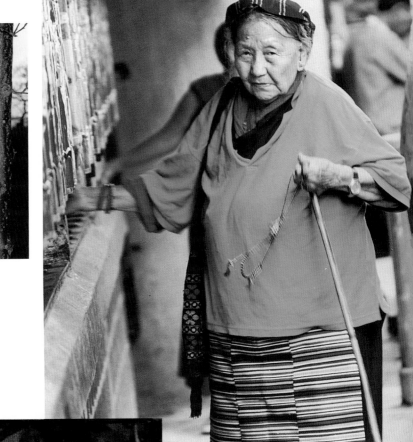

Photography has helped
me admire nature's magic
and realize the grace of life
in the present.

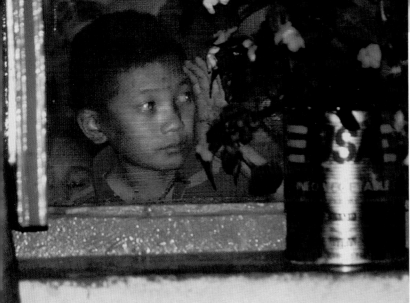

I was quite taken by the enduring spirit of this woman who
has survived so much and still
dreams of returning someday to
her homeland in Tibet.

I photographed this Tibetan
boy at an orphanage in India.
He nearly froze to death weeks
before as he fled on foot
through the Himalayas, and
to him the tin can bearing the
letters USA was a symbol of
freedom and hope.

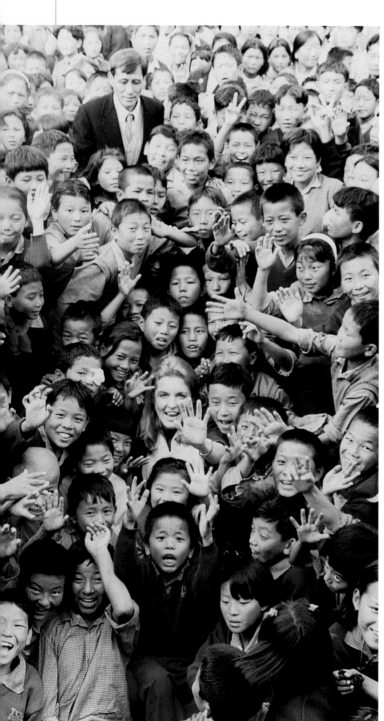

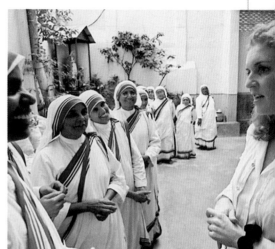

The grace and dignity so evident in
these nuns is matched by the
incredible strength and courage
which they draw upon while caring
for Calcutta's outcast and dying.

Everywhere I go in the world,
I'd like to see children treated as if
they are the center of our universe.

perience more fatigue than someone who ate 1,000 calories' worth of nutrient-rich foods and got a moderate amount of exercise. So it's the approach that may be the problem, not the effort to lose weight.

After all, research has found that losing weight—if you're overweight to begin with—can actually decrease fatigue and increase vim and vigor. There's no question that toting around extra pounds can be tiring, and that's because it's an added source of stress and strain for your body. Shedding excess body weight, on the other hand, can make it more comfortable for you to move through daily life, sleep more soundly, and boost your self-esteem, which can certainly help in the energy department. In a study at Tufts University School of Medicine and the Center for Clinical and Lifestyle Research in Shrewsbury, Massachusetts, eighty overweight women between the ages of 20 and 49 were randomly assigned to a twelve-week weight-loss program that included moderate to vigorous physical activity, 1,100 to 1,400 calories' worth of food per day, and weekly meetings, or to a control group. After twelve weeks, those in the intervention group lost significantly more weight than the controls had, which isn't surprising. What's interesting is that the intervention group also experienced marked improvements in several measures of quality of life, including their ability to function physically, their sense of vitality, and their mental health. In other words, they began to feel more upbeat physically and psychologically after losing weight.

The message: don't play the "how low can you go" game. When you cut your calorie intake too dramatically, your body interprets this as a threat and goes into starvation mode, slowing down all bodily functions to conserve energy. This can make you feel downright sluggish—and sabotage your weight-loss efforts. If you want to lose weight, stick with a reasonable daily calorie intake—such as 1,200 calories per day or more—and try to shed pounds slowly but steadily. Not only will this approach improve your odds of losing body fat and keeping it off, it will also help you keep up your energy level, which can only enhance your likelihood of staying with the plan.

When you make the shift from grabbing what's convenient to thinking in terms of what will give you good-quality energy, potato chips and doughnuts become less appealing. On the other hand, whole-grain carbs, lean protein, and colorful fruits and vegetables become more appealing. Eating for energy isn't about forbidding certain foods or depriving yourself of what you truly crave. It's about considering what you can eat that will help you have strength, stamina, and staying power as you go about the activities of your daily life. It's about making smart choices, rather than severely restricting them. But it's also about eating moderate amounts of lots of different foods—even small portions of those that have a relatively high fat or sugar content without feeling guilty about it.

It's a back-to-basics approach, with the focus largely on how food can benefit your body. This runs contrary to the way many people eat nowadays. They're so preoccupied with noshing on the run during a hectic day or preparing foods that cater to their kids' palates or eating foods that give them comfort that they don't give a thought to selecting foods that will give them lots of energy and help their bodies perform optimally. It's no wonder, then, that the obesity rate continues to climb—at this point, one in three U.S. adults aged 20 and over are obese and one in two are overweight—and approximately 51 million Americans will wind up going on a diet this year. Yet while most people consume more fat and protein than they should, they still manage to fall short in their recommended intakes of many important nutrients.

According to a recent report from the U.S. Department of Agriculture, many Americans, particularly women, are not getting enough of important vitamins such as B-6 or E or minerals such as calcium, magnesium, iron, and zinc. In fact, less than 25 percent of American women aged 20 and older consume diets that provide 100 percent of the recommended daily amounts of calcium, magnesium, and zinc. And while the USDA Food Guide Pyramid recommends that adults consume three to five servings of vegetables and two to four servings of fruit each day, only 41 percent of people are meeting their veggie quota and only 23 percent are consuming enough fruit. What this means is that many people are cheating themselves of a healthful diet—and top-notch fuel.

## The Core Components of Energy

When it comes to the nutritional cornerstones of energy, there are three primary players—carbohydrates, proteins, and fats—which are called macronutrients. The majority of foods people eat contain more than one of these macronutrients—pizza contains all three, for example—as well as vitamins and minerals, which are called micronutrients. Many foods also contain water, fiber, and phytochemicals (plant-based substances that have disease-fighting powers).

Many popular diet books would like you to believe that your body's ability to produce and use energy is rather fragile, that it depends on a precise ratio of macronutrients. But that's just not so. For example, few bodily processes are as tightly regulated as are the ups and downs of blood sugar. Insulin, a hormone that regulates the level of glucose in the blood, and glucagon, a hormone that stimulates the breakdown of glycogen (or stored carbohydrates) into glucose, work continuously to keep your blood sugar level within a narrow range. Small fluctuations in blood sugar are a normal part of glucose metabolism, and while there are a lot of theories linking low blood sugar to symptoms such as weakness, headache, and lethargy, these don't always hold up when they're subjected to scientific scrutiny.

## Carbohydrates and the GI Index

As far as readily available energy goes, carbohydrates are your body's best friends. For one thing, they provide direct energy for your brain, central nervous system, and muscles in the form of glucose (aka blood sugar), which can be burned (or oxidized) for running errands or a 10-K race or stored as glycogen for later use. Carbohydrates also supply energy to the body indirectly after they've been converted to starch or fat. You may have been taught that carbohydrates are categorized as either simple or complex—with simple being the low-quality choice and complex being the superior choice. But the classification of carbohydrates is more complicated than that. It's true that simple carbohydrates are sugars, whether they're from table sugar or the sugars in fruits or certain vegetables. But complex carbohydrates—which are found in whole-grain cereals, pasta, bread, legumes, and many vegetables—are also sugars, only in this case they're long chains of connected sugar molecules (some of which are easily broken down, others of which are virtually indigestible). Indeed, even complex carbohydrates are digested and metabolized in quite different ways, according to emerging research. This is one reason why the way carbohydrates affect blood sugar can't be predicted by whether a carbohydrate is simple or complex.

The newer thinking shows that different foods affect blood sugar in varying, but predictable, ways. Some foods cause a substantial and rapid rise in blood sugar, with a slow, prolonged return to its original level. Other foods cause only a modest increase in blood sugar, followed by a faster return to the baseline. These differences have led to the development of the glycemic index (GI), a system that ranks foods according to their effect on blood sugar levels.

While the concept behind the GI is universal, several ranking systems exist. The most accepted system compares what happens to blood sugar after a person consumes a particular food to consuming the same amount of white bread. Using this system, white bread has a GI of 100, glucose tablets are 137, and an apple is 54. Other systems rank foods from 0 to 70 or rate glucose tablets as 100.

Regardless of the specific numbers used, foods are considered to be high GI if they raise the baseline blood sugar substantially and/or for a prolonged period of time. Low-GI foods, by contrast, do not cause much of a fluctuation in the blood sugar. It's not easy to guess a particular food's GI. Suprisingly, a sweet potato has a lower GI than a white potato and carrots have a higher GI than many candy bars. (In Chapter 3, you'll find a table with the GIs of many common foods. There are also several books and Web sites with GI lists. It's important when using a combination of these references to know what the reference food is—such as white bread or glucose tablets—so that accurate comparisons can be made.)

The glycemic index is not always easy to put into practice, however. How quickly your blood sugar rises depends on the quantity of food you consume, your personal sensitivity, and what else you eat or drink with a particular food. After all, most people consume more than a single food at a given meal, which skews the GI picture. Besides, some carbohydrate-rich foods that have a high GI—such as carrots and watermelon—also provide plenty of health benefits in the way of fiber, vitamins, minerals, and phytochemicals. (Keep in mind: when choosing produce, the more vividly colored fruits and vegetables tend to contain more nutrients and health-protective phytochemicals.)

Your best bet may be to think of the glycemic index as a useful tool to guide many of your carbohydrate choices. The idea isn't to completely avoid foods with a high GI but to try to select foods with a low GI as often as possible. Or you could aim to include a low-GI food with every meal to help balance out the GI equation. Or you could replace higher-GI foods made from refined grains—bagels, white bread, and crackers, for instance—with lower-GI choices that are higher in fiber—whole-grain breads, barley, and the like. Choosing more foods with a low GI may help you achieve a steadier flow of energy and avoid the sudden cravings that can trigger overeating.

Aside from the fact that they're quickly converted into a usable form of energy, relying on carbohydrates as your primary dietary source of fuel—regardless of their GI— carries another advantage: it allows protein to fulfill its important role as a building block in cell growth and repair. If the body's supply of blood sugar begins to dwindle, stores of protein and fat step in as energy sources. But in order to metabolize fat efficiently, your body needs some carbohydrates, which is a problem if they're not available; in that case, your body enters a state of ketosis, which can cause health problems for some people.

# Importance of Dietary Fat

Fats are often perceived as a dietary foe, but they do have their place in an energy-boosting diet. While it's true that a high-fat diet can increase your risk of heart disease and some forms of cancer—not to mention adding unwanted pounds—some dietary fat is actually needed by the body. Why? Because it performs a plethora of essential roles, from making hormones and cell membranes to ensuring proper growth in children to promoting the absorption of fat-soluble vitamins such as A, D, E, and K to making eating more pleasurable by adding flavor and texture to foods. Dietary fats also help supply a significant portion of the energy that keeps your metabolism humming efficiently; plus, stored body fat can be converted into energy when your body runs low on carbs.

Not all dietary fats are created equal, though. While numerous reputable health organizations acknowledge that eating a diet that derives 30 percent or less of its calories from fat can stave off killer diseases such as heart disease, stroke, cancer, and diabetes, the type of fat also matters. After all, there are good fats such as unsaturated fats, found in olive and canola oils, corn and sesame oils, nuts and fatty fish, which reduce harmful LDL cholesterol. The most unhealthy fats are the saturated kind, found in meats and dairy products, and trans fatty acids, which are found in many margarines, French fries, and commercial baked goods; both of these types increase the risk of heart disease.

For the sake of your health, less than 10 percent of the day's calories should come from saturated fats and trans fatty acids; whenever possible, substitute unsaturated fats in place of saturated fats or trans fatty acids. Ounce for ounce, all of these forms contain the same number of calories—which happens to be more than double the calories that are found in the same amount of carbohydrates or protein. That's one reason why a high-fat diet can quickly lead to weight gain. What's more, a high-fat meal can leave you yawning and sluggish because it takes your body longer to digest fats. So those are two more good reasons to limit your fat intake.

# Protein—The Body Builder

Protein, as previously mentioned, is the body's major building material for the brain, muscles, connective tissues, skin, hair, nails, blood, and immune system. It is composed of amino acids and is essential to metabolic activities, tissue growth and maintenance, wound healing, the transport of nutrients, and many other vital bodily functions. (The very word "protein" is derived from the Greek word *proteios*, which means "of prime importance.") When it comes to energy, however, protein isn't a top provider: when the body's carbohydrate stores become depleted—if someone is eating too few calories or a very-low-carbohydrate diet, for example—protein can be broken down to supply the body with energy in the form of glucose. Normally, the protein will come from dietary sources, but if not enough is available it will come from the body's lean tissues, such as muscles, which is not what you want to happen. (You want to preserve all the lean muscle you can!)

Yet even though protein is so essential for so many bodily functions, many people consume more dietary protein than they need. The average healthy adult needs about .8 gram of protein for every kilogram (or 2.2 pounds) of ideal body weight. This means that a woman whose ideal weight is 130 pounds needs about 47 grams of protein per day—an amount that is easily achieved by eating a few ounces of meat, fish, or poultry, some dairy foods, and a variety of grains, cereals, fruits, and vegetables (all of which contain some protein).

Contrary to what many popular diets claim, there is no carb-protein-fat ratio that's ideal for everyone. A healthy range might consist of 50 to 60 percent of total calories from carbohydrates, 20 to 30 percent from fats, and the remainder from protein. For maximum energy, a general recommendation is to include some of each macronutrient in a meal. If you're trying to upgrade your energy level, you may want to adjust the ratio of carbs to protein, depending on the meal, while dividing your calories fairly evenly among your three primary meals (be sure to leave some leeway for snacks). For breakfast, you could strike a balance between the two macronutrients by having peanut butter on a bagel, cheese melted on toast, cereal with 2 percent milk and fruit, or a poached egg with whole-wheat toast and a glass of orange juice. For lunch, you could tilt the balance slightly toward protein—while keeping your fat intake low—to enhance alertness and productivity in the afternoon: A chicken burrito or a tuna sandwich plus a piece of fruit and a salad would be good choices to keep your mental motor working efficiently. Dinner is another story: when the day's activities are beginning to taper off and you want to set yourself up for a night of sweet slumber, that's a good time to have a carbohydrate-rich meal—such as a stir-fry with vegetables over rice or pasta with a marinara sauce. For many people, carbohydrates promote a state of relaxation and make them drowsy, so eating a carbohydrate-rich meal in the evening may be a savvy energy-regulating choice.

## The Value of Vitamins and Minerals

It's a mistake to think only in terms of macronutrients, though, because a varied diet that's rich in different vitamins and minerals is also essential to high-octane energy. After all, a nutrient-packed diet keeps your body functioning efficiently, which indirectly

## STRESS-FORMULA SUPPLEMENTS: SHOULD YOU BUY THEM?

As our lives have become increasingly harried, it seems that more and more stress-formula vitamin and mineral supplements have begun to crop up on drugstore shelves. While there's nothing wrong with taking a multivitamin and mineral supplement as a form of nutritional insurance, these particular products won't do anything special to create a calmer, more focused you.

Not all forms of stress are alike, and the nutrient contents of these supplements are based on physical stress and exertion, not psychological stress. But the truth is, these products are marketed to people who are under emotional strain. So if you're worrying about whether you're going to make next month's mortgage payment, these supplements aren't going to help you. But if you've recently begun to clock twelve-hour days doing heavy construction, they may help fill in some of the nutritional gaps in your diet.

contributes to producing energy and releasing it. But certain nutrients play starring roles in the energy picture—and many people don't realize this. Here are some of the primary players:

### Iron

During the childbearing years, women are especially vulnerable to iron deficiency because of the blood loss that's associated with menstruation. In fact, a recent study from the University of Newcastle in Australia found that young and middle-aged women who had a history of iron deficiency in the previous two years had lower scores on measures of physical health, well-being, and vitality than those without such a history. Iron deficiency reduces the amount of hemoglobin in the blood and prevents it from delivering adequate oxygen to the body's cells; as a result, you may feel tired, irritable, sluggish, or exhausted after a minor physical effort such as walking up a flight of stairs. If you're feeling droopy and you suspect that you may not be getting enough iron, consider increasing your intake of red meat, liver, egg yolks, wheat germ, shellfish, and fortified cereals.

### B Vitamins

Even borderline deficiencies in the B vitamins—including folic acid, B-6, and B-12—can cause fatigue, malaise, apathy, depression, and loss of concentration. That's because folic acid is needed to make red blood cells; and vitamins B-6 and B-12 are especially important for maintaining proper brain and nerve function. You can get plenty of folic acid from spinach and other dark green, leafy vegetables, orange juice, navy beans, and wheat germ. Good sources of vitamin B-6 include cereal, bananas, spinach, sweet potatoes, and prunes. Meanwhile, B-12 can be obtained from red meat, eggs, fortified cereals, seafood, and dairy products.

## Potassium

Along with sodium, which is another electrolyte, potassium helps to regulate the body's fluid balance. It's also critical for proper metabolism and the transmission of nerve impulses and muscle contractions. If you get dehydrated or contract a gastrointestinal illness (with vomiting or diarrhea), your body's potassium reserves will be drained. A diet that's rich in fruits and vegetables usually provides enough potassium. If you suspect you're low in this essential nutrient, stock up on bananas, oranges, apricots, bran, potatoes, and beans.

## Magnesium

It's important for numerous chemical reactions in the body, including the production and release of energy, the transmission of nerve impulses, and proper muscle function. If you don't get enough magnesium, you're likely to feel fatigued. Fortunately, magnesium is available in a wide array of foods, including green leafy vegetables, whole grains, meat, fish, dried beans, nuts, seeds, and dairy products.

## Zinc

Not only does zinc improve muscle strength and endurance, but it also assists with the digestion and metabolism of carbohydrates, protein, and fat. It's also involved in the functioning of your nervous system and wound healing. Because this mighty mineral serves so many functions, a zinc deficiency can cause lethargy, poor appetite, and increased susceptibility to infection. Foods with a high zinc content include beef, lamb, oysters, yogurt, wheat germ, and fortified cereals.

## Calcium

Best known as the must-have mineral for maintaining healthy bone density, calcium also promotes muscle and nerve function, helps blood to clot, and reduces symptoms of PMS, including fatigue. Yet the vast majority of women don't consume enough calcium. If you don't like dairy products, good sources of calcium include canned salmon, turnip greens, broccoli, tofu, and fortified orange juice.

If fulfilling your quota of essential vitamins and minerals on a reduced-calorie diet seems like Mission Impossible, it may not be your imagination. The reality is, it's hard to get all the nutrients you need if you're consuming fewer than 1,200 calories per day. In that case, taking a supplement can help fill in the nutritional blanks in your diet and perhaps boost your energy. Look for a supplement that contains a broad range of vitamins and minerals with about 100 percent of the recommended daily value for most nutrients. But don't count on getting all the calcium you need from a multivitamin: It's too bulky a nutrient to fit in with all the others, so you'll need to take a separate calcium supplement.

# False Energy Boosters

Even if you're religious about eating a nutritious diet and popping a daily multivitamin, you could be squandering your energy in subtle ways with what you put in your mouth. When you're in the throes of an energy slump, what do you reach for? If you're like many women who feel as though they're perpetually overcommitted or crunched for time, your boosts of choice are likely to come in the form of caffeine, alcohol, or nicotine. But all of these will let you down, even if they pick you up initially.

Coffee can pep you up in the short term but drop you like a ton of bricks later. In moderate amounts, coffee or tea can increase alertness and concentration, lift your mood, stimulate your central nervous system, and improve your thinking ability and reaction time. But the energizing effects last only for up to two hours, at which point you're likely to return to a slump. Once you're truly hooked on coffee, you can also suffer withdrawal symptoms, including headaches and fatigue. If you drink too much coffee, you'd be wise to cut back gradually—by incrementally adding decaffeinated to your regular coffee.

If you typically feel emotionally spent in the evening, do you have a drink or two to help you unwind and restore your equilibrium? There's nothing wrong with having an occasional cocktail in the evening. But imbibing more than one or two too often is a mistake in the energy department for three reasons: one, because alcohol is a sedative, which means it will make you feel sleepier sooner than you normally would; two, because it can dehydrate you; and three, because it can compromise the quality of your sleep, possibly causing you to wake up during the night. (It's also full of empty calories—meaning that alcoholic beverages contain calories but few nutrients.) This doesn't mean you have to become a teetotaler, but it is wise to consume alcohol in moderation—meaning one drink per day for women, two drinks per day for men. It's also smart to have an extra glass of water for each glass of wine, beer, or spirits you imbibe to counteract the dehydrating effects of alcohol.

Nicotine is also a no-no in the energy department. Yes, it stimulates the central nervous system, so it may pep you up in the short term. But it will bring you crashing down before long. Not only does smoking impair your breathing—both during exercise and in everyday life—but it also compromises the delivery of oxygen to your body's tissues, which makes you feel fatigued. If you smoke, your best bet is to call it quits—once and for all. Your health will improve, and you'll have more energy and stamina.

These days, all sorts of products are available that promise pep in a package or effortless weight loss. Many of these pills, potions, teas, and concoctions contain ephedra (aka ma huang), guarana or other exotic-sounding ingredients. For many people, it's hard to resist the idea of revving up your metabolism, curbing your appetite, or jump-starting your energy just by swallowing a pill or drink. After all, these products are preying upon people who are looking for a quick fix for their energy crises or their weight woes. But it's unwise to buy into these claims. If these products do increase your pep, it's because they are stimulants, pure and simple. And for that reason they can be dangerous: ephedra is a controversial Chinese herb that has been linked with serious illnesses, strokes, and even deaths; guarana extract is a source of caffeine that can adversely affect those who are sensitive to caffeine—or have an additive effect if you're a java junkie.

## THE ULTIMATE ENERGY DRINK

Move over, energy drinks. Water's here—and it's here to stay. After all, it's the quintessential health and energy elixir. It's the most plentiful substance in our bodies, accounting for 50 to 75 percent of our weight, and the component that's most necessary for survival. Besides being essential to digesting, absorbing, and transporting vital nutrients, building tissue, and maintaining body temperature, good old $H_2O$ is needed by every cell in the body to perform its fundamental activities. Water also lubricates the joints, helping them move smoothly, and gently supports the lungs, spinal cord, and brain.

Yet even though water fulfills these myriad vital functions, many people don't consume enough of the stuff. They're walking around in a state of mild dehydration and—surprise, surprise—one of the first signs of dehydration is fatigue. Indeed, it's a mistake to wait until you're thirsty to hit the bottle, as thirst is not a reliable indicator of hydration. By the time the thirst mechanism kicks in, you've already lost 1 to 2 percent of the fluid in your body, which means you're mildly dehydrated. Even mild dehydration can make you feel tired or lethargic. What's the best gauge of whether you're drinking enough water? The color of your urine. If it's bright yellow, it's time to drink up. If it's pale yellow, you're probably well hydrated.

To make sure you're getting all the $H_2O$ you need, your best bet is to come up with a daily water plan, just as you do for your meals. If you're sedentary, aim for at least six cups of $H_2O$ per day, more if you're very active. Think about when you're going to drink, carry a water bottle with you, and increase your water intake by eating lots of soups, fruits, and vegetables. Make water your beverage of choice at meals (it's calorie-free to boot), and take a water break instead of a coffee break at work. To make water more appealing, you can add lemon or orange wedges or make a thermos of herbal (noncaffeinated) tea. Then drink to your health and vitality.

Indeed, some of these products may actually present stealthy threats to the health of those who take them. And there's no way of predicting who might have an adverse reaction; individual sensitivity to the ingredients varies dramatically from one person to the next. So it's a bit like playing supplement roulette. Often it's the combination of what you're taking with everything else in your life—how much caffeine you consume, what other drugs you take, whether you smoke, and so on—that can cause problems. But problems do occur: in fact, researchers at the University of California, San Francisco, recently reviewed 140 reports of adverse events related to the use of ephedra-containing diet supplements that were submitted to the Food and Drug Administration between June 1, 1997, and March 31, 1999. What they found is that 62 percent of the reactions were definitely, probably, or possibly related to use of the products; 47 percent of these involved cardiovascular symptoms such as high blood pressure, heart palpitations, rapid heart beat, stroke, and seizures; and 18 percent involved the central nervous system. The bottom line: you'd be smart to steer clear of these products and improve your eating, exercise, and lifestyle habits instead.

# Why Starving or Stuffing Yourself
# Can Sabotage Your Energy

Some people find that consuming large, heavy meals can weigh down their get-up-and-go, making them feel sluggish for several hours. What's more, large, high-fat meals place an added strain on your body: recent research suggests that eating a heavy meal can increase a person's risk of having a heart attack by ten times in the following hour. That's because after a heavy meal, the heart beats 20 to 30 percent faster and the power of each beat is harder than usual, which is an extra stress to the heart, according to study author Francisco Lopez-Jimenez, M.D., a cardiologist at Brigham and Women's Hospital in Boston.

## THE SKINNY ON SERVINGS

There's so much talk these days about the importance of exercising portion control and sticking to recommended serving sizes. But do you have any idea what a proper serving actually looks like? If not, you're hardly alone. When in doubt, it's always a good idea to weigh and measure your portion sizes. If that's not possible, you can often eyeball it by picturing servings of specific foods as the shapes of everyday objects. Here are some examples:

2 servings of bread = **two slices of bread = a videocassette tape**
2 servings of cooked rice or pasta = **1 cup = a tennis ball**
1 serving of fresh fruit = **1 cup = a baseball**
1 serving of veggies = **1 cup = a clenched fist**
1 serving of cheese = **1½ ounces = a pair of dice**
1 serving of cooked meat or chicken = **3 ounces = a deck of cards**
1 serving of fish = **3 ounces = one and a half cassette tapes**

When it comes to eating for sustainable energy, don't be afraid to tinker with your eating pattern. The key is to find an eating regimen that works for you. For many people, three meals per day suits them best but others may find that eating minimeals throughout the day helps them stay on an even physical and emotional keel, curb hunger, and stay energized for longer periods of time. Most people get hungry every four hours, so you could eat three square meals a day plus a couple of snacks or six minimeals. If you decide to try the minimeal approach, be sure to downsize your portions—by using a salad plate instead of a dinner plate, for example, or a coffee cup as a soup cup instead of a huge bowl. Whichever pattern you choose, you may want to divvy up your calories evenly throughout the day for more sustained energy. Chances are, you'll know within a couple of days if the new eating pattern suits you.

## Putting the Pieces Together

By now you've probably begun to recognize that choosing and eating the right foods can give you more energy—and help you lose weight. So from now on, strategy is in; winging it is out. This means you'll need to start eating smartly by consuming a variety of foods but concentrating on whole grains, veggies, fruits, and lean protein. It means you'll need to start limiting your fat intake and avoiding large, heavy meals. (Exercise portion control!) It means you'll need to start keeping your consumption of sugar, alcohol, and caffeine to a moderate level. And it means you'll need to join the breakfast club and start the day with a healthy morning meal. People who eat a substantial breakfast, as well as lunch and dinner, burn 5 percent more calories per day than those who skip breakfast, according to obesity expert C. Wayne Callaway, M.D., of George Washington University in Washington, D.C. Every extra calorie that's burned will help. Of course, eating smartly also means eating enough to provide your body with the energy it needs to perform all the activities that make up your jam-packed life.

Once you develop your personal energy-eating plan and you tune into how various meal patterns make you feel, you'll begin to discover the formula that revs you up and keeps you going. The only way to do this is through trial and error, and the only person who can do it is you. After all, you are the engine that drives your energy. So think of this as a way of devising your very own energy diet, one that offers an enormous payoff: more verve and vitality, greater stamina, and less exhaustion—plus a greater chance of achieving a healthy weight.

When it comes to fueling your energy with food and beverages, how savvy are you? To find out, answer these questions.

1. Which of the following breakfasts would be the most likely to jump-start your energy for the day?
   a. A bowl of oatmeal with low-fat milk and a banana
   b. A fruit salad and toast with jam
   c. Coffee with a multivitamin

2. How often do you generally have something to eat?
   a. Every three to five hours
   b. When I can no longer stand my hunger pains
   c. Whenever I get the chance to sit down to an uninterrupted meal

3. In the midst of a hectic day, which of the following lunch choices are you likely to make for lasting fullness?
   a. A bowl of lentil soup with a whole-wheat roll
   b. A turkey sandwich with mayo on multigrain bread
   c. A cheeseburger with fries

4. When you hit a midafternoon energy slump, which of the following are you most likely to use to keep yourself going?
   a. A small container of low-fat yogurt and an apple
   b. A cup of coffee and a cereal bar
   c. A small bag of reduced-fat chips and a diet soda

5. When cooking something that requires sautéing, which of the following are you most likely to use?
   a. Nonstick cooking spray
   b. Olive or canola oil
   c. Stick margarine or butter

6. If your stomach starts growling between meals and you feel your energy flagging, what do you do?
   a. Have a handful of trail mix or whole-grain crackers
   b. Wait ten minutes and see if the feeling goes away
   c. Tough it out until the next meal

7. Which of the following is the beverage of choice for keeping you energized?
   a. Plain water or seltzer with a twist of lemon or lime or a splash of juice
   b. A glass of orange juice
   c. Coffee, tea, or an energy drink

8. If you want to settle down in the evening and set yourself up for a good night's sleep, what might you want to have for dinner?
   a. Whole-wheat pasta topped with shrimp and steamed vegetables
   b. Broiled fish, a salad, and a baked potato
   c. A large serving of meat loaf and mashed potatoes

9. How can you tell if you're drinking enough water?
   a. Your urine is pale yellow
   b. You drink water with every meal
   c. You hardly ever get thirsty

10. What are the most important vitamins and minerals for adequate energy?
    a. All of them are essential to keeping your body running smoothly
    b. Iron, the B vitamins, and zinc
    d. The antioxidants: A, C, and E

Now Let's see how you did.

Mostly As: you have got a firm grasp of the effect that your eating habits can have on your energy. Keep these facts in mind—and strive to find new ways to put them to use in your life.

Mostly Bs: you have got a good sense of the basics but you may be squandering your energy in subtle ways. Which means that your energy IQ could use a little tune-up; you'll get it from the following pages.

Mostly Cs: you need to bone up on the relationship between eating and energy. But don't worry: reading this book will help you gain a sense of how to make smarter choices and incorporate them into your life.

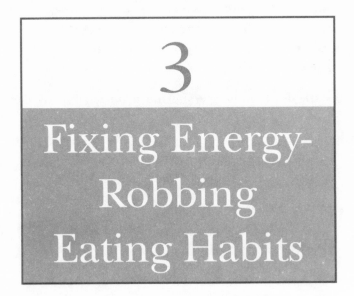

# 3
# Fixing Energy-Robbing Eating Habits

Imagine you are about to marry the man of your dreams, and on the day of your wedding you are exhausted and almost blinded by a migraine headache. Of course I was nervous, but my love for my future husband was more than enough to conquer my wedding jitters. I think my pain had little to do with nerves and everything to do with a terrible diet I'd been following for several months to make sure I'd fit properly into my wedding gown. I speak often of this diet, one on which I subsisted on red meat and citrus juice. Water, vegetables, or any other food ways not permitted, and even though I knew such a diet was unhealthy, I was able to justify sticking with it: feeling terrible was the price I had to pay for being over-weight. Yet the headaches and exhaustion persisted after my honeymoon, and I was hardly surprised when my doctor told me that this bizarre diet was, in effect, still taking its toll on my entire system. As I began eating normal food again, I was rav-enously hungry and craving the creamy, fatty, and savory dishes I'd forced myself to give up. I rebounded from that diet by overeating everything I'd missed. No surprise as to what happened next: the weight I'd lost—and then some—came right back.

Within weeks of our being married, Andrew was shipped off on active naval duty, leaving me on my own and unprepared for my new role. Before my marriage, I shared a small walk-up flat with my best friend, Carolyn, and back then I managed to avoid cooking as much as possible. I liked to eat, but I knew little about nutrition and less about whether my eating habits were healthy or not. I was good at making sacrifices after an indulgence, though. I was quite good at skipping meals or fasting; you see, the "pain for pleasure" dieting model made perfect sense in my mind.

As if adjusting to the pressures of public life were not enough, my chaotic approach to eating wreaked all kinds of physical and emotional havoc. I can remember days when I'd have to face a full day of official engagements on the equivalent of an empty gas tank. In the early days I seemed tireless in my work, but when my weight was creeping up I'd often skip breakfast entirely and only pick at lunches and dinners when I was in public. It's no wonder there were days when I felt faint and found it hard to concentrate. No wonder I'd break down and binge in private late at night on the stash of goodies I'd squirreled away in our quarters at Buckingham Palace.

Fast-forward to today: Now I'm busier than ever. I'm quite proud of the fact that at 42 years of age I manage to keep going as if I were still in my twenties, rarely running out of steam. And if I do, I'm able to rejuvenate myself quickly. What's different nowadays is my approach to eating: it's smarter, even strategic.

I have a new love in my life these days, and he has four legs. I am mad about Bobbu, an extraordinary show jumper of whom I'm now owner. Bobbu is already quite a star in Europe, and I believe that with proper care and consistent training he'll soon be a world-class competitor. My horse has all the advantages of an excellent diet, vigorous

## 5 NATURAL ENERGY BOOSTERS

1. Wheat grass juice is not particularly tasty, but just a tiny glass provides me with a bit of "mule kick" when I need it.

2. Ground gingerroot steeped in hot water makes a tea that's soothing and awakens the senses.

3. Aromas such as peppermint and basil are thought to have invigorating effects.

4. Pump up your lunchtime salad with some protein, such as strips of turkey breast or some fava beans.

5. Get moving. Break that sluggish feeling by standing up and taking a vigorous walk. Even a fifteen-minute jaunt around the office or down the block can leave you feeling revitalized.

exercise, and regular visits to the vet, and it shows in his feisty demeanor and energy in the ring. Had we neglected any of these factors, Bobbu might never come close to reaching his potential. Now I apply the very same principles to myself.

On busy days, it pays to think ahead about when and what you'll eat. There are times on business trips when a hotel's kitchen does not serve breakfast until 6:00 A.M—just as I'm getting into a car heading off to my first appointment. A phone call ahead to the hotel manager may be all it takes to request an early breakfast order or at least to make sure that a simple meal is prepared for me the night before. It helps me to pack along some single-serving portions of dried fruit or a raisin-and-nut mix, which is a simple and healthy energy booster perfect for a late morning snack. Last year I had speaking engagements for Weight Watchers in Des Moines in the morning and Omaha in the afternoon. No air service connects the two cities, so we had to drive nearly two hours between engagements. I packed a light but satisfying box lunch with cubes of savory meats, cheeses, baked crackers and bread sticks, and some whole fresh fruit. On arrival I was rested and raring to go onstage before 1,500 Weight Watchers members, leaders, and staff. I spoke for nearly an hour, then did a string of interviews and ended our visit with a tour of a corporate wellness site before heading out for our flight to Denver.

Again, for me it's about adapting my scheduling to what works for keeping my energy soaring. As I mentioned, the one thing in my life that I find can truly sap my energy is traveling. Air travel can be chaotic, and even short flights can prove exhausting. But I try to see the positive side: I think of the time I'm in my seat as pri-

## THE ART OF GRAZING

"Grazing lets you eat when there's no time for a meal. Skipping meals leaves me tired and increases the likelihood that I'll overeat. If I'm on a tight schedule, I'll pack some nutritious foods that I can nibble on to keep up my energy and keep hunger at bay. In addition to bottled water, I may pack fresh vegetables and fruits, bite-size pieces of cheese or lean meat such as baked ham or chicken breast, baked crackers, and perhaps one or two low-fat dips."

vate downtime to relax and regroup. Short hops may offer nothing more than a chance to kick off my pumps and replenish myself with a bottle of mineral water. Meals served on longer routes may not be to my liking, so I find that ordering a vegetarian selection or fruit plate in advance keeps me from feeling sluggish later. In fact, I only nibbled at my salad during the flight to Denver, knowing that I'd be sitting down to dinner with my team later that evening. In a busy workweek, I prefer a dinner consisting of a leafy salad, broiled fish, and a serving of steamed vegetables such as asparagus or spinach. I usually limit myself to one glass of wine and finish dinner over a hot cup of herbal tea, which relaxes me before bed.

I do get blasts of energy in other ways that have nothing to do with food. Sometimes I need to remove myself temporarily from the circuslike atmosphere before one of my personal appearances. Believe it or not, I still get nervous about speaking to large groups, and it helps me to take a few moments by myself to breathe slowly and focus on how very lucky I am. Of course I get a huge lift from the smiling eyes of people who come out to see me, and I deeply appreciate their kindness because I know the hours of waiting in line can be just as draining for them.

You've probably heard a lot about power bars and energy drinks that rev you up. These may be fine for an occasional quick pick-me-up, but remember that no one food or drink can make you feel vital and energized. The way to truly boost your energy is to follow a long-term, well-balanced diet that draws on a variety of food sources so the building blocks of good nutrition come together like a wall that can hold up against the stresses of everyday living.

# Food, Energy, and You

As the saying goes, "You are what you eat."—That's especially true when it comes to energy. Treat yourself to the right mix of nutrients and plenty of water all day long, and you'll probably be humming along in high gear. Stuff yourself with the wrong foods—or deprive yourself of essential fuel when you are hungry—and you might suffer a body and brain energy drain. Pump your body with essential vitamins and minerals—without overdoing them, of course—and you're likely to feel vibrant and zestful. Deny your body the nutrients it needs to function efficiently, and you're likely to feel weak and listless. Your energy level can go either way, depending to some extent on how you eat. It's a simple matter of dietary management—or mismanagement, depending on which approach you end up taking.

The good news is, jump-starting your energy can begin with modifying the way you eat. You can create meals that will perk you up instead of dragging you down if you give the subject a little forethought. You might find, for example, that eating a protein-rich lunch—such as a grilled chicken sandwich—can provide you with a boost in mental energy during the afternoon. Or you might find that eating a high-carbohydrate meal—such as pasta primavera—can make you feel soporific in the evening. Or you might discover, with a little experimentation, that having a midafternoon snack that ranks low on the glycemic index (GI)—a cup of low-fat yogurt and a pear, for example—can help you stay charged for a late-afternoon workout.

People respond differently to different foods and eating styles, so it's important to find what works best for you in terms of meal frequency and meal composition. Since few of us consume meals that consist solely of a single food, the key to using food to regulate your energy flow may be to tinker with the ratio of carbohydrates to proteins in any given meal, as well as aiming for a balance between high and low GI foods. Don't just practice this approach on an as-needed basis, though; it needs to become a habit, day in and day out, if you want to tune in to the effect that different foods have on your personal energy level. After all, consistency plays a vital role in the energy equation.

# Following the Food Guide Pyramid

With few exceptions, the foods and beverages that are most likely to provide you with premium energy are the same ones that will help you manage your weight. Indeed, the best way to ensure that your battery stays well charged is to consume a healthy diet that's full of whole grains, fruits, and vegetables, as well as some lean protein and dairy products. Following the USDA Food Guide Pyramid can help you in this respect: After all, the base of the pyramid—which contains the stuff that should make up the largest part of your diet—is the bread, cereal, rice and pasta group, which is the top dietary source of high-octane complex carbohydrates. Depending on your calorie intake and how active you are, the recommendation is to have between six and eleven servings from this group per day. A serving equals one slice of bread, half an English muffin or bagel, ½ cup of pasta or rice, one tortilla, or one ounce of ready-to-eat cereal. One criticism that has recently been voiced by Walter Willett, M.D., chairman of the department of nutrition at the Harvard School of Public Health, and others is that the pyramid overlooks the notion that the types of carbohydrates you eat can make a difference. After all, different foods can cause blood sugar to rise or fall at varying degrees and speeds, and different carbohydrates are richer or poorer in fiber and important nutrients. The best carbohydrates to use as the foundation for a healthy diet, they contend, are derived from whole grains, beans, and other less refined sources. But the pyramid makes no distinction about quality in this respect.

On the second level of the pyramid are fruits and vegetables, which are good sources of vitamins, minerals, and dietary fiber. Again, depending on your calorie intake and activity level, the recommendation is to have two to four servings of fruit and three to five servings of vegetables each day. A serving equals one large kiwi or one medium-size apple or banana, ¾ cup fruit juice, about 5 large strawberries, ½ cup raspberries or blueberries, or 9 dried apricot halves. A serving of veggies, on the other hand, consists of ½ cup of cooked vegetables, 1 cup of raw leafy greens, about 8 baby carrots, 1 medium baked potato or ear of corn, 1 cup of bean soup, or ¾ cup vegetable juice. All vegetables are healthy—assuming you don't add lots of fat in the preparation—but starchy vegetables such as corn, peas, and potatoes tend to be denser in calories than their nonstarchy counterparts—asparagus, broccoli, peppers, spinach, and the like—so you may want to make the majority of your veggie servings nonstarchy.

As you make your way up the pyramid, the serving recommendations shrink, mainly because these foods are from the protein group and tend to be naturally higher in fat. And the truth is, most people consume plenty of protein and fat as it is. It's recommended that you have two to three daily servings from the milk, yogurt, and cheese group, and an additional two to three servings from the meat, poultry, fish, beans, eggs, and nuts group. A serving from the dairy group consists of 1 cup of milk or yogurt or 1½ ounces of cheese, whereas a serving from the meat category equals 2 to 3 ounces of lean beef or pork, 2 to 3 ounces of cooked fish or poultry, ½ cup cooked dry beans, 1 egg, or ⅓ cup nuts or seeds.

At the peak of the pyramid is the fats, oils, and sweets food group, which you should consume sparingly.

Not only does the Food Guide Pyramid help you follow a diet that's good for your health, it can also help you boost your energy. After all, with the pyramid, you'll obtain the bulk of your calories from carbohydrates, the body's primary source of energy. You'll make moderate selections of protein and use fats in small amounts. (Just as the pyramid doesn't distinguish among the GIs of foods, however, it doesn't distinguish among different types of fats; as previously mentioned, it's best to stick with unsaturated fats as much as possible.) By using the pyramid, you'll have variety, balance, and moderation in your diet—and you'll likely feel healthy and vibrant. The key to creating sustainable energy—and losing weight, if that's your goal—is to eat enough of the right foods but not so much that you feel weighted down or sluggish.

# FOOD GUIDE PYRAMID
## A Guide to Daily Food Choices

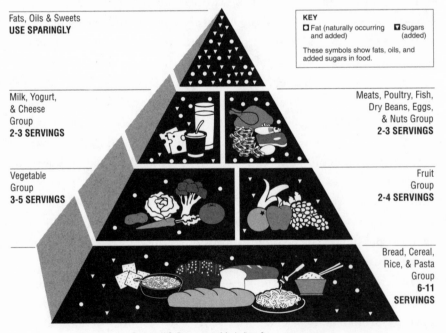

Fats, Oils & Sweets
**USE SPARINGLY**

KEY
□ Fat (naturally occurring and added)   ■ Sugars (added)
These symbols show fats, oils, and added sugars in food.

Milk, Yogurt,
& Cheese
Group
**2-3 SERVINGS**

Meats, Poultry, Fish,
Dry Beans, Eggs,
& Nuts Group
**2-3 SERVINGS**

Vegetable
Group
**3-5 SERVINGS**

Fruit
Group
**2-4 SERVINGS**

Bread, Cereal,
Rice, & Pasta
Group
**6-11
SERVINGS**

Source: U.S. Department of Agriculture &
U.S. Department of Health and Human Services

# The Food Guide Pyramid and the GI Index*

Since the Food Guide Pyramid doesn't account for the glycemic index, chances are you won't know which carbohydrate choices are likely to make your blood sugar rise quickly or in a more sustained fashion. Part of the challenge with the glycemic index is that it's not intuitive; it's simply too difficult to guess where on the GI spectrum a particular food might fall. That's why it's smart to familiarize yourself with some general trends in the GI, rather than worrying about specific numbers.

Here's how the choices stack up in terms of the glycemic index.

## In the Bread, Cereal, Rice, and Pasta Group

HIGH GI: Bagels, waffles, most breads, hamburger buns, cornflakes, oat cereal, instant oatmeal, rice, crackers, croissants, doughnuts, commercial muffins

MEDIUM GI: Pumpernickel bread, toasted muesli, bulgur, linguine, and most other white pastas

LOW GI: 100% bran cereal, rice-bran cereal, barley-kernel bread, barley, vermicelli

## In the Vegetable Group

HIGH GI: Carrots, beets, baked potatoes, French fries, corn, sweet potatoes

MEDIUM GI: Peas, baked beans, pinto beans

LOW GI: Black beans, chickpeas, navy beans, kidney beans, lentils, soybeans, split peas

## In the Fruit Group

HIGH GI: Bananas, fruit cocktail, mango, kiwi, pineapple, raisins, watermelon, orange juice

MEDIUM GI: Oranges, grapes, pineapple juice, grapefruit juice, apple juice

LOW GI: Apples, dried apricots, cherries, grapefruit, pear, plum, fresh peaches

## And in the Dairy Group

HIGH GI (ABOVE 70): Ice cream, tofu frozen dessert

MEDIUM GI (55 TO 70): Custard

LOW GI (BELOW 55): Milk (skim and full fat), chocolate milk, low-fat yogurt with fruit

*Adapted from "International Tables of Glycemic Index," American Journal of Clinical Nutrition, 62 (suppl.) (1995): 871S–890S.

# Getting More Satisfaction

There's no denying that it's nearly impossible to feel energetic when hunger is gnawing at your belly. Indeed, veteran dieters are all too familiar with one of the cardinal frustrations of trying to lose weight: not feeling full or satisfied after a low-calorie meal. Wouldn't it be liberating if you could concentrate on choosing foods that put your hunger to rest, instead of obsessing about every calorie that crosses your lips? Well, you can. The latest thinking among some diet experts is that one of the best strategies for managing or losing weight is to select foods with a high satiety value—meaning that they're filling and satisfying—and naturally low in calorie density—meaning that you can eat large quantities for relatively few calories.

After all, satiety influences how much food you consume in a given sitting as well as how soon you'll feel like eating again and how much you'll eat at that time. So increasing the satiety value of your meals is like getting more bang for your nutritional buck. By building meals around foods that offer satisfaction for fewer calories, you won't feel physically or psychologically deprived, and you'll have plenty of energy to sustain your activities for several hours. This will help you peel off unwanted pounds. Opinions vary regarding whether carbohydrates or proteins are more satiating, but some nutrition experts now believe that energy density is crucial to the satiety issue: If you can eat a larger quantity of a particular food for relatively few calories—because it is low in calorie density—you'll have a better chance of feeling satisfied longer. In fact, high-fat foods are the most problematic when it comes to weight management because they are easily overeaten: not only are they highly palatable and high in calories, but they also have a low satiety value compared with carbohydrates. So you wind up eating more than you'd intended.

Indeed, a study by researchers at the University of Sydney in Australia ranked various foods according to their ability to provide satiety: They fed dozens of common foods to forty-one people who weren't dieting and two hours later allowed participants to eat as much as they wanted from a buffet. This way, the researchers could measure how well the previous foods, based on 240-calorie portions, banished hunger. The ten most filling foods turned out to be boiled potatoes, steamed cod fillets, cooked oatmeal, oranges, apples, wheat pasta, broiled lean beef, baked beans, grapes, and whole-wheat bread. Interestingly, the ten least filling foods were croissants, iced chocolate cake, cinnamon sugar doughnuts, a chocolate-caramel candy bar, roasted peanuts, strawberry yogurt, potato chips, vanilla ice cream, muesli cereal, and white bread. What the satiating foods have in common, for the most part, is a high fiber and water content—plus low calorie density. What most of the least satiating foods have in common is a high fat content and high calorie density.

# Satiety and Weight Loss

The secret of losing weight without sacrificing satisfaction may be to increase the volume of food you consume while lowering the calorie density. This way you can trick your body into feeling fuller for longer, have plenty of energy, and shed unwanted pounds. Research has found that people tend to consume the same volume of food over the course of a week, even if what they actually eat varies considerably from day to day. In a recent study at Pennsylvania State University, for example, researchers found that both lean and obese women consumed a similar volume—but not weight—of food daily, even when the fat content and calorie content varied from one day to the next. So if you can increase the volume of the food you eat without increasing the calorie content, you'll have plenty of energy and lose weight.

Sound like the impossible dream? It's not. One way to consume fewer calories without compromising satiety is to increase the volume of your food without increasing its calorie count—by adding water or air. Some foods—such as fruits, vegetables, low-fat milk, cooked grains, fish, beans, and soups—are relatively low in calories and naturally have a high water content. Eating more of these foods can help you slim down and feel buoyant. This way, you can actually eat more while consuming fewer calories than usual—by having 1¼ cups of grapes instead of ¼ cup of raisins, for the same 100 calories, or by having chicken rice soup instead of a chicken rice casserole, for example.

Recently, researchers at the Conservatoire National des Arts et Métiers in Paris examined the soup sipping habits of five thousand Parisians and found that those who were considered "heavy consumers" of soup—defined as having soup five or six days out of every six—consumed fewer calories at dinner than those who occasionally or rarely had soup. What's more, women who were heavy consumers of soup were more likely to have a body mass index (BMI) under 23—they were slim, in other words—than those who weren't. The moral of the study: having water- or broth-based soup with a meal can help you fill up for fewer calories, which will likely lead to weight loss.

Another way to increase the volume of the food you eat is to choose items that are rich in fiber or packed with air (think puffed cereals or extra-whipped smoothies). Indeed, researchers from Penn State University found that increasing the volume of a food—in this case, by adding more air to a yogurt smoothie—caused a group of men to subsequently consume 12 percent fewer calories at lunch because they felt that much fuller. The key to cutting calories effectively is to strive for comfortable fullness that lasts—without compromising your energy.

If you want to increase the volume and satiety level of your meals, here are some savvy high-energy swaps to make throughout the day:

## Breakfast
INSTEAD OF: A croissant with butter

TRY: A heaping bowl of oatmeal with chopped apple or pear

## Lunch
INSTEAD OF: A grilled cheese sandwich and potato chips

TRY: A steaming bowl of lentil vegetable soup with whole-grain crackers

## Snack
INSTEAD OF: A doughnut or cookies

TRY: A big bowl of microwave popcorn

## Dinner
INSTEAD OF: Fried chicken or a hamburger, French fries, and a piece of cake

TRY: Flank steak or broiled fish with boiled or baked potatoes and green beans, and a bowl of grapes

## MORE ENERGY-BOOSTING MEALS

Planning and preparing energy-regulating meals doesn't have to be rocket science. It's really a matter of picking and choosing the right foods from the right food groups, as you've seen. Here are several additional suggestions to get you through the day with plenty of physical and mental energy—when you need it most.

**ENERGIZING BREAKFASTS:** Scrambled eggs with mushrooms and zucchini and a piece of toast; half a multigrain bagel with light cream cheese and smoked turkey; a mini–bran muffin, low-fat yogurt, and a peach or plum.

**PEP-INDUCING LUNCHES:** Couscous salad with chicken and veggies; a sandwich on whole-grain bread with grilled vegetables and cheese; a tortilla wrap with turkey, peppers, spinach, and a low-fat dressing.

**RELAXING DINNERS:** A stir-fry with vegetables and shrimp over brown rice; a chicken breast, a baked potato, and steamed asparagus; pasta tossed with garlic, vegetables, and grated mozzarella cheese.

# Smart Strategies for Different Situations

Wouldn't it be amazing it you could create your own personal antifatigue diet? Well, you can. But in order to do that, you'll need to fine-tune your eating habits so that you'll gain plenty of energy when you naturally tend to droop and be able to do more in each day and also lose weight (if that's your goal). Since the timing and content of what you eat can have a dramatic effect on your get-up-and-go, this means that you can use food to your advantage by tinkering with your diet in such a way that it addresses your personal energy deficit and helps you navigate your way over the stumbling blocks. What follows are four common scenarios with smart strategies on how to feed your body for peak energy.

## Situation: You Have PMS and You're Feeling like a Basket Case All Day Long

**Solution:** Women often experience more energy swings than usual in the premenstrual phase of their menstrual cycles, and some women are especially sensitive to these fluctuations. Plus, many women experience intense cravings for certain foods such as chips or chocolate. When PMS is raging, the solution is to drink lots of water and to eat minimeals that focus on low-GI foods every two to three hours throughout the day. Some women find this can help them battle the fatigue, food cravings, mood swings, and headaches that may crop up before their period makes its monthly appearance. Consider noshing on fruit-and-yogurt smoothies or whole-grain crackers with mozzarella cheese every few hours to keep cravings in check.

## Situation: You're Getting By on Too Little Sleep

**Solution:** There's no getting around the fact that this means you're not getting the rest your body needs to meet the demands you're facing. It's a bit like pushing a car down the road instead of sitting inside and driving it. Sooner or later, you're going to have to replenish those lost hours of shut-eye. In the meantime, you might try eating smaller, more frequent meals—every three hours. And aim to eat more unprocessed carbohydrates (such as fresh fruits and vegetables) and low-fat protein (such as chicken or fish) to boost alertness.

## Situation: You Tend to Feel like a Zombie by 2 or 3 P.M.

**Solution:** Believe it or not, this midafternoon energy slump is due to the body's normal circadian rhythms. (That's why it is the custom in some countries to take a siesta around this time of day.) Fortunately, you can counteract the drop somewhat by taking a catnap or a walk and then having an energy-boosting snack—such as a small amount of trail mix or a fruit-and-yogurt smoothie—with a large glass of water afterward. Don't rely on caffeine to pull you through this dip; the temporary jolt will be fleeting and could leave you feeling even draggier later.

## SNACKING DONE SMARTLY

The next time hunger strikes between meals, don't be caught off guard. Be prepared—by keeping these smart, energy-boosting choices on hand. Here's a shopping list with ten quick ideas for refueling in the middle of the day.

1. Whole-grain crackers or brown rice cakes spread with peanut butter
2. A piece of fruit with half a cup of low-fat yogurt
3. A couple of fig bar cookies and a glass of skim milk
4. A small box of raisins with a stick of low-fat cheese
5. Baby carrots with low-fat bean dip
6. Half a whole-wheat English muffin spread with light cream cheese
7. Half a whole-wheat pita filled with lettuce, tomato, cucumber, and a dollop of hummus
8. A hard-boiled egg with two sesame breadsticks
9. A baked apple with cinnamon, a tablespoon of chopped walnuts, and a spoonful of low-fat vanilla yogurt
10. A glass of tomato or vegetable juice, a slice of low-fat cheese, and two whole-grain crackers

### Situation: You Don't Have Enough Energy to Exercise

**Solution:** Exercise does require extra energy, so it's wise to fuel up and drink up ahead of time. To prevent your energy from waning halfway through a workout, have a carbohydrate-rich snack with a little protein at least an hour before exercising. A few snacks that should do the trick: a small apple with a slice of cheese, yogurt with fruit, or half a small whole-grain bagel with peanut butter. Be sure to drink 16 ounces of water an hour before your workout and 6 to 8 ounces every twenty minutes during the session.

# The Ten Commandments of Eating for Energy

Could it be that your own weight-control efforts are sabotaging your energy? It's possible. Countless women routinely commit dietary blunders that drain their energy and set them up to fail at losing weight. It shouldn't be that way. While it can be challenging to plan healthful meals when your plate of responsibilities is already overflowing, it can be done. All it takes is a knowledge of the basic tenets of eating for energy with an infusion of motivation and mindfulness. With that in mind, here are ten rules for using food to tip the energy balance in your favor:

COMMANDMENT 1: *Thou Shalt Not Skip Meals.*
If you want to start the day on the right foot—namely, with a spring in your step and an upbeat attitude—eat breakfast as well as regular meals throughout the day. Otherwise you'll wind up feeling lethargic, and you'll probably get overly hungry—and possibly set yourself up for overeating—later in the day. Just as you wouldn't set off on a trip when your car's gas tank registers empty, you shouldn't jump into your day without refueling after the previous night. For optimal energy, your best bet is to eat a morning meal within three hours of awakening. Ideally, choose something that combines protein and carbohydrates and includes a fruit serving. It could be peanut butter on a bagel, cream cheese on toast, cheese pizza, an energy bar, or old favorites like cereal, milk, and fruit or a poached egg with whole-wheat toast and a glass of orange juice.

COMMANDMENT 2: *Thou Shalt Not Have a Heavy Midnight Snack.*
It's not that noshing late at night is more likely to lead to weight gain than eating at any other time of day. But the foods people tend to eat in the hours between dinnertime and bedtime—ice cream, cookies, chocolate, chips, and so on—are often high in fat and calories, which can cause extra pounds to accumulate. Plus, consuming a heavy meal late in the evening can give you middle-of-the-night indigestion, which can wreak havoc on your slumber. As a result, you may awaken the next morning feeling dead tired. If you can't kick the snacking-before-bed routine, your best bet is to have a light dinner and to later have a sleep-friendly snack such as a small cup of cereal with milk or a cup of chamomile tea and some graham crackers.

COMMANDMENT 3: *Thou Shalt Not Be Reckless with Caffeine.*
Gulping cup after cup of coffee to keep yourself going won't fire up your energy continuously. Yes, the caffeine can perk you up for an hour or two, but drinking too much can

make you feel wiped out later—or dependent on the stuff. And because it alters brain chemistry, similar to the way adrenaline does, it can heighten your reaction to stress and interfere with sleep, both of which can make you feel exhausted in the end. That's why it's smart to limit your caffeine intake to three servings—the amount in a 5-ounce cup of coffee or tea—or less per day.

## POWER IN A PACKAGE

An astonishing array of products—from energy bars to energy beverages—has hit the market, promising instant pep and power. Do they deliver? Will they rev you up? Or are they nothing more than glorified candy bars or soft drinks in fancy wrappings?

The truth is, there's nothing about them that's special for energy, other than the fact that they provide the body with calories. But so do other foods. Most of these products do contain vitamins and minerals, as well as carbohydrates, which places them higher on the snack hierarchy than candy bars. Many also contain soy products, decaffeinated green tea extract, flaxseed, and other ingredients that may appear to promote good health but may not be present in sufficient quantities to do much of anything. By the same token, a few of these products also contain potentially dangerous herbal additives such as ephedra, so be sure to read the label carefully. That way, you'll know what you're actually getting in each bite.

Of course, the main advantage of these products is convenience: you can grab them and stash them in your purse or briefcase for a quick on-the-go snack. The energy bars are likely to work better in terms of providing sustainable energy because they are digested more slowly than the liquids are and hence have longer staying power. But they aren't free of calories—they contain anywhere from 170 to 300 per bar—so be sure to factor this into your calorie-intake budget.

COMMANDMENT 4: *Thou Shalt Not Eat the Same Foods Day After Day After Day.*

In their quest to lose weight, many people start rigid diets, in which they eat the same foods day after day and wind up getting bored with those foods. Not only will this lead to taste-bud fatigue, which can set you up for overeating in desperation, but it will deprive your body of a variety of nutrients that are necessary for optimal energy. What to do: Plan menus ahead of time that offer variety and appeal to different senses. Consider buying a low-fat ethnic cookbook or two. Make it a rule to eat one food you've never tried at least once a week. When eating out, order something healthy that you've never had before. Eating can be an enjoyable adventure—without leading to overindulgence. Besides, flexibility can be a dieter's best friend. In a recent study at Louisiana State University in Baton Rouge, researchers examined the dieting strategies of 223 men and women, half of whom were significantly overweight. What they found was that flexible dieting was associated with the absence of overeating, whereas calorie counting and conscious dieting were associated with overeating and increased body mass.

COMMANDMENT 5: *Thou Shalt Not Obsess About What to Eat.*
It's good to be mindful about what you're eating for the sake of weight control, especially since we live in an environment of amazing abundance, particularly when it comes to food. But it's quite another thing to take dietary restraint to an extreme. Indeed, many women expend enormous amounts of mental energy thinking about calories, fat grams, good foods versus bad foods, and how much of any given item it's safe to eat. Besides being psychologically exhausting, exercising excessive dietary restraint—consciously restricting your food intake severely in order to prevent weight gain or encourage weight loss—can be taxing on the body. In fact, a recent study at the University of British Columbia in Vancouver found that women who scored high on measures of cognitive dietary restraint secreted higher levels of cortisol in their urine; this is noteworthy because cortisol is a marker of stress that may have a detrimental effect on bone health. Previously, this same group of researchers had found that restrained eaters experienced short luteal phases of the menstrual cycle, which caused their cycles to be infertile. In addition, research has found that restrained eating can make people more vulnerable to overeating when under stress: in a recent study at University College London in the United Kingdom, researchers found that people who were restrained eaters were more likely to eat more calories when they experienced high levels of work stress, including long hours on the job; unrestrained eaters, by contrast, were not vulnerable to stress-induced eating under these conditions.

COMMANDMENT 6: *Thou Shalt Not Fast to Cleanse Your System.*
Fasting may help you drop a few pounds quickly, but it'll be mostly water weight and some muscle, neither of which is healthy or desirable in the long run. Losing water weight can lead to dehydration and electrolyte imbalances, both of which can sap your energy. And you don't want to lose muscle in the course of dieting because the more lean muscle you have, the faster you'll burn calories all day long; after all, it's muscle that revs up your me-

tabolism. And the idea that fasting cleanses out your system is pure hogwash: when your body is deprived of food, chemicals called ketones can gradually build up; these chemicals tax the kidneys unnecessarily, which can be dangerous to your health and give you bad breath, to boot. If you want to jump-start your diet, a better approach is to eat lightly, exercise vigorously, and drink lots of water.

COMMANDMENT 7: ***Thou Shalt Not Pile Your Plate with Too Many Choices.***
Variety may be the spice of life, but overdoing it could also mean the downfall of your diet. In a recent review of thirty-nine studies, researchers at the University of Buffalo in New York found that food consumption generally increases when more variety is provided in a given meal. This may be because under these conditions people don't get tired of the taste of a particular food and put down their forks as a result; instead, they simply move on to another food and continue eating. Which can lead to overeating and a feeling of sluggishness. Of course, this doesn't mean your meals should consist of only one food. It just means you should offer yourself a limited array of choices in any meal. One palatable way to do this: Fill three-quarters of your plate with fruits, vegetables, and whole grains, and the remaining one-quarter with lean protein and fat sources. When it comes to choosing fruits and veggies, keep in mind: the darker the color, the more health-protective properties it's likely to have.

COMMANDMENT 8: ***Thou Shalt Not Eat on the Run.***
Not only will you miss out on the sensory enjoyment of eating—as well as a chance to catch your breath in the midst of a hectic day—but you could set yourself up for making poor food choices and for overeating. After all, if you eat too quickly, you're likely to end up eating more—whether it's now or later—for two reasons: because you'll miss out on the sensory quality of the food, and because it takes twenty minutes for the brain to register that you're full. A better idea: Give yourself at least twenty minutes to sit down, eat slowly, and pay attention to what you're eating—how it tastes, how it feels in your mouth, how it makes you feel, and so on.

COMMANDMENT 9: ***Thou Shalt Not Deny Your Cravings.***
If you have a real hankering for chocolate and you try to quench it with an apple, chances are you just won't be satisfied. Instead, you might continue to eat around your craving—adding some crackers or cereal and then something else—and wind up eating more in the long run. Not only will this approach pack in lots of extra calories, but it may make you feel full and sluggish as well. You'd be better off having the one true thing you really crave

to begin with but in a small serving. If you have a cup of chocolate sorbet or a few choco-late kisses, for example, you'll get the taste you yearn for without filling up and weighing yourself down.

**COMMANDMENT 10:** *Thou Shalt Not Forget to Enjoy Your Meals.*
Yes, eating is a utilitarian task in the sense that you do it to provide your body with the fuel it needs to function well. But eating is also a sensory experience that can be filled with pleasure—if you let yourself savor your food, that is. So while you're aiming for a bal-ance of nutrients, try to create meals that also provide a balance of textures, tastes, and aromas. A few tricks: a dash of avocado, garlic, sesame or walnut oil goes a long way toward enhancing flavor without adding lots of fat and calories; so do fresh herbs and spices and flavored vinegars. Stock your pantry with salsas, hot sauces, and other savory seasonings that will increase the flavor quotient of your food without adding many calo-ries. You might also consider giving your favorite dishes a makeover—by learning new ways of preparing them with less fat, for example, or by taking a healthy gourmet cooking class. Of course, you can still enjoy your favorite foods, even if they're high in calories, so long as you do so in moderation. After all, no food should be taboo. If you exercise mod-eration in all your choices and keep an eye on the big picture, your meals can be enjoy-able, varied, healthful, and energizing—without compromising your waistline.

**QUIZ:** *What's the Energy–Weight Loss Equation?*

Are you fueling your energy or making it fizzle with your eating habits? Likewise, are you supporting your weight-loss efforts or sabotaging them? Believe it or not, the two issues are not mutually exclusive. To find out how you're doing, read the following questions and then mark them True or False.

1. To lose weight and keep up your energy level, it's best to stick with a prescribed num-ber of balanced meals per day.
2. If you want to shed pounds without losing energy, stick with at least 1,200 calories per day.
3. If you're trying to lose weight, you should eat breakfast only if you're hungry.
4. One of the best ways to consume fewer calories with a meal is to start with a bowl of broth-based soup.
5. If you're aiming for a steady blood sugar level, your best bet may be to choose foods from the high end of the glycemic index.

6. You should eat slowly because it takes the brain twenty minutes to register fullness.
7. If you obsess about what you eat, you're less likely to overeat.
8. Eating a combination of protein, carbohydrates, and fat will provide you with energy for several hours.
9. Fat is just as dense in calories as carbohydrates and proteins are.
10. You can increase the volume of the foods you eat without increasing your calorie intake.

Scoring:

| | | |
|---|---|---|
| 1. | T = 1 | F = 2 |
| 2. | T = 2 | F = 1 |
| 3. | T = 1 | F = 2 |
| 4. | T = 2 | F = 1 |
| 5. | T = 1 | F = 2 |
| 6. | T = 2 | F = 1 |
| 7. | T = 1 | F = 2 |
| 8. | T = 2 | F = 1 |
| 9. | T = 1 | F = 2 |
| 10. | T = 2 | F = 1 |

Now add up your score and see how you fared.

**17–20 points:** Congratulations! You've got the know-how that it takes to fill yourself with high-octane energy and lose pounds. Now the challenge is to put it into practice on a consistent basis.

**14–16 points:** You're headed in the right direction—namely, toward boosting your vitality and slimming down—but a few gaps in your knowledge could trip you up along the way. Time to fill them in.

**10–13 points:** It looks as if you need a refresher course in the basics of eating for energy. Review this chapter—and the previous one—and you'll be in a better position to fuel your body for high energy and weight loss combined.

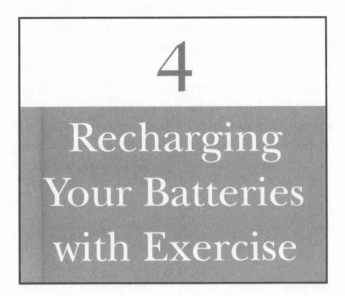

# 4

# Recharging Your Batteries with Exercise

When I was a girl, I had boundless energy. Growing up on a farm, I loved nothing better than riding with my ponies. In fact, I dreamt of being a show jumper one day. I was sporty all through my school years, and even when I was having weight problems I never lost my athletic edge. I think it was due to the fact that I love sports, such as alpine skiing, and I took pride in my skill as an equestrian. I could rise to the occasion of a ski holiday or a weekend ride, but I was hardly in peak condition. My sporadic bursts of physical activity would be followed by aches and fatigue. Just as important, though, was the fact that being out of condition was affecting me in my everyday life, as well.

Being athletic and competitive as I am, you'd think I'd adore working out in the gym, but I do not. When I was twelve years old, my parents sent me to Hurst Lodge, a school noted for its ballet, thinking it was an ideal finishing school for their tomboy daughter. I was lucky to be admitted, but it proved a bit of a disaster. While I had the kind of explosive energy that made me excel on the playing field, I hated the precise movements and the repetitive nature of studio workouts.

If you hate the idea of going to a gym, please don't let that stop you from finding an exercise regime you can enjoy. There are lots of options and activities that you can do at home. Because of my crazy schedule, Josh, my trainer, has devised a workout that can be done in a gym or at my home. We don't work out in a room full of expensive equipment, although I do have a stationary bicycle, which simulates riding on all kinds of different terrain. Then the workout is fairly basic: stretches, resistance exercises and use of hand weights. In my case, working with a trainer helps me get the most out of my workout time. Josh's routines really challenge me, and what I like is that he adapts them to my energy level on any given day. He has taught me the value of variety and continuity in my fitness routine.

Whether or not you have a trainer, please don't cheat yourself of personal time for fitness. The physical and psychological benefits of regular exercise, doing whatever workout you choose, will not only make you stronger, it will enhance many parts of your life.

Of course, being fit is not contingent on special equipment, either. Walking can be a fantastic workout requiring no special tools other than a pair of good walking shoes. I think it's fabulous that many communities now have walking clubs, so your workout can become a social affair. Also, if you fancy kickboxing or a step workout but classes aren't for you, exercise videos or fitness shows on television can offer a solo workout with the guidance of a top professional. In other words, the only thing that can stop you from getting in top shape is yourself.

A number of years ago, I was invited by a top fashion magazine to be photographed for one of its covers. Of course I was flattered, yet I felt some trepidation about stepping into the realm of supermodels. My initial hesitation turned to anxiety on the day of the shoot as the studio stylists and fitters went about squeezing me into the narrow evening gown they'd picked out. It would have been a lovely dress had I been skinny, but I was cringing as the seamstress complained about my hips being too wide for it. Meanwhile the hairstylist was busy gluing long locks of red hair to my scalp to create the latest "do." It would have been a fantastic look on a girl half my age, but all that extra hair just wasn't me. As you might expect, after hours of fussing, I stepped in front of the camera bearing little resemblance to my real self. Weeks later I received a call from the magazine's editor, who politely informed me that I would not be on its cover after all. She explained that I looked "weighty," tired, and sad in my shots (who wouldn't after what happened at the shoot?), and the news hurt me in a deep and personal way. After we hung up, I paused for a few moments to consider how I felt about all this. I was healthier than I'd ever been, and I had no illusions about being a fashion model. I liked the fact that I now felt good about myself and about the way I looked, so I decided then and there that I would not let losing a magazine cover take that away from me.

To look at all the buff models in fashion magazines, it's easy to conclude that fitness equates with being ultrathin. There's no denying that working out can enhance your shape, but most of us will never be shaped like fashion models, no matter how thin we become. Instead, I like to focus on the invisible benefits. For instance, physical activity, along with a good diet, is essential to cardiovascular health. I was delighted when the American Heart Association asked me to help promote heart health among women. Heart disease is the number one killer of American women, but the good news is that there is plenty a woman can do to prevent heart disease, much of it revolving around regular physical activity as well as a heart-healthy diet.

As a mother, I am also keenly aware of the fact that what I do in terms of living a healthy lifestyle for myself also sets a good example for my girls. It's alarming that so many children today are inactive, opting to play video games or watch TV instead of playing in the yard or trying out for sports. I make it a point to fill up the girls' leisure time with all kinds of physical activities that I know they enjoy. Like all children, though, they sometimes need Mum's prodding to get up and moving. I recall one rainy weekend last spring when Beatrice and Eugenie seemed to be milling about with no particular outlet for their nervous energy. They thought I was quite mad when I finally suggested they take their ponies out for a run. "In the rain?" they asked, looking amazed at the very idea of it. "Come on," I said, slipping into my slicker and rubber boots, and soon the three of us trudged off to the stable for what turned into hours of active fun. If you have children, or even grandchildren, taking time out to be together teaches them to be active their whole life—and at the same time it can keep you feeling young, too.

## FEELING OVERWHELMED

"If you are feeling overwhelmed, it's probably time to reassess your priorities and your commitments. I've organized my life under an 'umbrella' that has three main categories: Family, Me, and Work. I keep lists for each, and when I'm getting overloaded I see which things must be done now, which can wait, and which can be delegated to someone else to handle. The process of reassessing these lists daily or at least weekly helps me separate out what I need to do."

# Exercise and Energy

Wouldn't it be great if scientists could come up with a single remedy that could provide you with more energy almost instantaneously? One that would make you feel better, stronger, and more zestful as soon as possible? Well, in this case, scientists won't need to spend long hours toiling in the laboratory because such a treatment already exists. It doesn't come in pill form; nor is it an elixir you can simply swallow. It's exercise—and it really does work wonders at banishing fatigue, improving mood, enhancing your health, slowing the aging process, and combating stress. Granted, the notion that expending energy through exercise can actually give you more energy may sound paradoxical. But it makes sense: regular exercise improves physical fitness, and a fit body produces and uses energy with less strain than an unfit one does. A fit body also fatigues less easily, which means it has greater reserves of stamina and endurance. In other words, a fit body has energy to spare.

So why haven't more of us become hooked on this miraculous energy enhancer? Partly because of the lifestyle conundrum that many of us face these days: How to reap the energy-boosting effects of exercise when you haven't got the energy to exercise in the first place? While it's true that exercise does use energy in the sense that it burns calories or fuel, physical activity usually generates more palpable energy than it uses up. Usually a moderate workout makes you feel invigorated and vibrant. Yet excuses about not having enough energy to exercise can create a vicious circle: without the energy-boosting effects of exercise, the fatigue cycle simply continues, and week after week, you still don't feel as though you have the energy to embark on—or stick to—a workout regimen. As a result, working out probably gets relegated to the bottom of your "to do" list, and it simply becomes another item that rarely gets done.

Indeed, it seems as though we're in the midst of an epidemic of inactivity: approximately 25 percent of adults in the United States do not engage in any physical activity whatsoever in their leisure time, according to the latest statistics from the Centers for Disease Control and Prevention. Meanwhile, only 22 percent of adults in the United States participate in regular, sustained physical activity, which is defined as any type or intensity of activity that occurs five times or more per week for 30 minutes or longer per session. And about 15 percent of U.S. adults say they perform regular, vigorous physical activity, which is defined as exercise that is performed at thirty percent or more of a person's cardiorespiratory capacity (or $VO_2$ max) three times per week or more for at least twenty minutes per session.

Nevertheless, despite these relatively low exercise participation rates, research has found that year after year, vowing to start exercising regularly ranks among the most common New Year's resolutions people make. But only a small percentage of people actually follow through on this good intention to the point where it becomes a habit. Indeed, research has found that half of people who start an exercise program drop out within three to six months.

## The Mind-Body Benefits of Exercise

If the thought of exercising brings a grimace to your face, replace it with a grin. It's worth doing whatever it takes to get yourself moving—whether this includes bargaining with yourself or bribing yourself, if need be—because the potential payoffs of exercise are enormous. Not only will working out regularly help you manage your weight and lower your risks of all sorts of life-threatening diseases—including heart disease, many forms of cancer, type II diabetes, osteoporosis, and others—but it can also provide you with a surge of energy that can last for hours.

How does exercise work its energy-boosting magic? Let's count the ways. For starters, it gets your heart pumping faster, sends air flowing briskly through your lungs, contracts your muscles and improves their tone, and promotes the flow of blood and oxygen throughout your body, thereby carrying vital nutrients to your cells. Exercise also revs up your metabolism, which can help you burn calories at a faster rate even when you're not working out, particularly if you increase your muscle mass. Regular aerobic exercise and muscle-strengthening exercise can also promote better-quality sleep, which can make you feel more rested and refreshed the next day. And, of course, it can help you lose weight by burning extra calories.

The cumulative effect of all these benefits is a body that uses energy more efficiently. As a result, you'll be able to do more physical activity with less stress and strain on your body, which will make that particular activity feel that much easier—and leave you with extra energy for other activities on a given day. The energy-boosting effects of exercise are so powerful that they have even proven to help people who are undergoing chemotherapy, which is notorious for inducing severe, relentless, debilitating fatigue. In a recent study at Oregon Health Sciences University and the Oregon Cancer Center in Portland, for instance, researchers found that regular low-to-moderate-intensity exercise significantly reduced fatigue for women who were receiving chemotherapy for breast cancer. Moreover, the length of their workout sessions and the intensity of the exercise had an inverse relationship to their fatigue levels, meaning that longer exercise sessions and exercise at a higher intensity each had a stronger impact on easing fatigue. (In this particular study, the energy-boosting effect lasted for only one day.)

Just in case all these benefits aren't reason enough to make you a reformed sofa spud, consider this: study after study has found that exercise has the power to ease depression and improve mood, which can promote energy and a positive take-charge approach to life. There's good scientific evidence that exercise does work its wonders on the mind, as well as the body. After all, exercise alters brain chemistry—namely, by sparking the release of mood-enhancing endorphins and increasing levels of the feel-good neurotransmitter serotonin, which can leave you with a feeling of calm energy. Of course, exercise also improves blood and oxygen flow throughout the body and brain, which can reduce tension and increase alertness. In fact, in a recent study of 156 adults with major depressive disorder, researchers at Duke University Medical Center in Durham, North Carolina, discovered that exercise alone was as effective in relieving depression as the use of antidepressants and as effective as the combination of antidepressants and exercise were. What was even more surprising is that those in the exercise group had lower relapse rates after ten months than did those in the medication group.

Further down on the scale of emotional distress, exercise can also help you bust out of a garden-variety bad mood. In a series of studies at California State University, researchers evaluated the success of various strategies that more than four hundred people commonly used to beat bad moods, boost energy, and reduce tension. What they found was that exercise appears to be the healthiest and most effective way people regulate their own moods and energy levels; relaxation techniques came in second.

In addition to exercise's direct mood-enhancing effects, believing that you are actually capable of exercising regularly seems to confer a confidence-boosting benefit that can then enhance your mood: research from the University of Illinois at Urbana-Champaign has found that when people believe they are highly fit and able to succeed at particular physical activities, they are more likely to reap emotional benefits from exercise. In this case, it appears that believing leads to the feeling. In another study, this same group of researchers found that previously sedentary middle-aged adults experienced a significant improvement in self-esteem and physical self-worth over the course of a twenty-week exercise program. These emotional changes can, in turn, lead to a rosier outlook and a more upbeat attitude toward life—to a boost in psychological energy, in other words.

Last but not least, going to the gym or out for a walk carries another hidden—but incredibly important—benefit: it's time away from the ever-ringing telephone or doorbell, the demanding kids, a cranky boss (or family member), and other sources of energy-draining stress. It's time spent doing something positive and healthy for you. Indeed, it's a form of self-maintenance and self-enhancement that is bound to have an energizing effect on your body and mind.

# The Three Facets of Physical Fitness

More often than not, a fit body has plenty of energy for the activities of daily living because a fit body can perform everyday movement with less stress and strain—and because a fit body is better able to deliver oxygen throughout the body and remove waste products. Moreover, when you become fit, your breathing ability improves, as does the ability of your muscles to use oxygen and generate force. The sum total of these improvements is that you really do have energy to spare. It's like having a full—and bigger—tank of gas before embarking on a long trip: your energy-building capacity will have increased, and you'll have plenty of fuel in reserve. This is why an amount of exercise that might feel difficult when you first start working out will gradually feel easier as you continue with it over a period of weeks. The way to derive all these energy-boosting benefits is to embark on an exercise program that encompasses the three facets of physical fitness: aerobic exercise, muscular strength training, and flexibility.

## Aerobic Exercise

Aerobic exercise—continuous physical activity that uses large muscle groups and is intense enough to condition the heart and lungs—is a powerhouse in the energy equation, largely because it enhances the oxygen-toting capabilities of the blood as well as airflow through the lungs. During aerobic exercise such as walking briskly, running, swimming, biking, cross-country skiing, rowing, skating, or stair climbing, your body increases its consumption of oxygen and continuously delivers it, along with nutrients, to your muscles and cells. The word "aerobic" literally means "with oxygen," and aerobic exercise refers to any repetitive activity that can be done for a long enough period of time and at a hard enough intensity that it moderately challenges your heart and lungs; that's why it's often called cardiorespiratory conditioning. The latest guidelines from the American College of Sports Medicine (ACSM) recommend aerobic exercise three to five days per week for twenty to sixty minutes at a stretch. Fortunately, aerobic benefits usually begin to come fairly quickly after embarking on a regular exercise program, which means that what might feel difficult today will feel considerably easier within a few weeks.

In order for exercise to be truly aerobic and produce a conditioning effect, you'll need to work out at your target heart rate—between 60 and 80 percent of your maximum heart rate. (To calculate your maximum heart rate, subtract your age from 220—this number estimates your maximum heart rate in beats per minute. Now, multiply the resulting number by .6 to gauge the lower limit of your target zone and by .8 to figure out the upper limit.) You can tell if you've reached this target zone by taking a break and immediately checking your pulse on your wrist: Count the number of beats in fifteen seconds, then multiply the result by four to figure out your heart rate in beats per minute.

If you'd rather skip all the mathematical calculations, that's not a problem. Simply gauge the intensity or difficulty of the activity you are performing by rating it on a scale of 0 to 10, with 0 being an intensity of "nothing at all" and 10 being "very, very hard." This is called a Rating of Perceived Exertion, and it reflects how hard you feel you are working when exercising. What you should be striving for is "somewhat hard"—somewhere between four and eight on a ten-point scale. How hard is somewhat hard? You should be able to carry on a conversation while you exercise, but you shouldn't be able to sing your favorite radio jingle.

## Strength Training

As far as the energy equation goes, strength training—which is also known as resistance training and refers to performing specific exercises against resistance or gravity—is especially important for stamina (also called muscular endurance). After all, preserving and strengthening your muscle mass will allow you to generate more strength and force in a particular physical feat with less effort, which means that your muscles will gain greater endurance and tire less easily. In addition, building muscle revs up your metabolism because lean muscle burns calories at a faster rate during and after exercise than body fat does. In other words, from a metabolic perspective, you may have a "hotter" body: pound for pound, muscle burns 35 to 50 calories per day compared to only 2 calories per day for body fat. So if you gain lean muscle through strength training, you'll also gain a metabolic boost, which can lead you to experience a reduction in body fat even if your weight doesn't change. In fact, in a recent study at Arizona State University, researchers found that performing resistance exercises fired up the metabolisms of the moderately trained women for up to two hours after the workout. In another study, researchers at the University of Maryland found that a strength-training program increased people's resting metabolic rate by 7 percent after six months.

Now for the bad news: Lean muscle mass tends to decrease with age (a condition called sarcopenia), dragging down your resting metabolic rate with it. This is one reason why people naturally tend to gain body fat as they get older: if they don't cut their calorie intake to compensate for the metabolic slowdown they've experienced, they'll put on fat—

an average of half a pound to one pound per year through adulthood. Being dedicated to strength training—whether you choose to move against gravity by doing crunches and push-ups, create resistance by lifting free weights, use machines such as Nautilus or Cybex, or perform exercises with rubber tubing or Dyna bands—can offset some of this age-related muscle loss. It can also prevent bone loss, improve your posture, prevent back problems, and help you lose weight. And it can help you look better by toning and sculpting your muscles, making them more defined in the process. Plus, muscle is more compact than body fat is, which means that you could actually drop a dress size simply by adding lean muscle and shedding body fat, even if the number on the scale doesn't budge.

The latest American College of Sports Medicine (ACSM) exercise guidelines call for strength training two to three days per week but not on consecutive days since muscles need ample time to recover from the stress you're placing on them. One set of 8 to 12 repetitions of 8 to 10 exercises that target all the major muscle groups—in the arms, shoulders, chest, abdomen, back, hips, and legs—will do the job as far as building and maintaining muscle mass goes. This may sound time-consuming, but it can be done in thirty minutes or less—time that is well spent. After all, research has found that doing one set of 15 strength-training exercises just two times per week can lead to a gain of three to four pounds of lean muscle within two to three months.

## Flexibility

Flexibility is the third component of a good exercise program, yet it's probably the most neglected one. But with flexibility, too, more is better, which means it's just not possible to stretch too often. After all, flexibility is important for helping you move your joints and muscles safely through their full range of motion. In fact, recent studies suggest that flexibility training in the form of stretching exercises may actually enhance muscle performance. Not only will increased flexibility allow you to perform everyday activities more comfortably, it will also ease muscle tension and decrease your risk of getting injured. This is especially important as you get older, because with the passing years, muscle fibers and tendons tend to shorten and tighten, which can restrict your range of motion (and hence your flexibility). When this happens, your posture won't be as erect as it used to be, you'll walk and move around more stiffly, and you'll find it harder to bend over to tie your shoelaces. All of these changes can make you feel awkward and constricted in your body.

You can gain flexibility by doing yoga, tai chi, or stretching exercises. Or you can incorporate stretching into your aerobic workouts after you've warmed up for five to ten minutes by walking or biking at a gentle pace, for example; at that point, you can take a short break to slowly stretch all the major muscle groups—in the calves, thighs (including the quadriceps and hamstrings), butt (aka the glutes), pelvis, lower back, arms, and shoulders. Be sure to move slowly and extend a stretch to the point where you feel a modest tension in a particular muscle and hold the position for twenty to thirty seconds; don't bounce, and don't push a stretch to the point of pain. The ACSM now recommends that you perform stretching exercises at least two to three days per week.

# The Exercise Prescription

When it comes to giving yourself more vim and vigor, aerobic exercise is the single most important form of exercise because it helps generate energy for prolonged periods of time and improves the way your heart, lungs, and muscles function in continuous movement. Strength training counts, too, though, especially when it comes to improving your muscles' ability to generate strength and force and when it comes to boosting your muscular endurance. And enhancing your flexibility will improve your energy indirectly—by helping you move more smoothly through a wider range of motion and reducing your risk of injury in everyday activities as well as exercise.

Despite the energy-producing hierarchy of these various forms of exercise, all three are important to bolstering your get-up-and-go because they have an additive beneficial effect on each other. When combined, the three forms will give you a complete fitness package that can boost your stamina, strength, and elasticity—and thus your sense of vitality. Although it may seem like a tall order just to carve out the hours to do all this exercise—especially if you're strapped for free time and overwhelmed by life's pressures, as many people are these days—it doesn't have to be. The trick is to find creative ways to combine these forms of exercise or to squeeze them separately into a hectic schedule.

## Creating a Regimen

How should you put the pieces together? By breaking the fitness components down to their essential parts, then fitting them together in a way that suits your personal schedule. If you plan to exercise first thing in the morning, for example, you might decide to go for a brisk walk or jog for thirty minutes on Monday, Wednesday, Friday, and Sunday before having breakfast; make a concerted effort to stretch after your walk, and you will have sneaked in a little flexibility training. Then, on Tuesdays and Thursdays, you could spend half an hour doing strength-training exercises, followed by more stretching. When you break a recommended exercise prescription down into its basic elements, then arrange them in a way that makes sense for your life, it's much easier—and less time-consuming—to fit it all in than it probably seemed at first blush. If you're just not up to the task of devising your own program, don't worry: we've taken the guesswork out of creating an all-encompassing fitness plan by providing a four-week walking program that also incorporates strengthening and flexibility-enhancing moves in Chapter 5.

What's important with this or any exercise plan is to start slowly—at a pace that feels reasonable and comfortable to you—and to build up to more challenging workouts. That way, you'll be able to safely increase your stamina, lower your risk of injury, and increase the odds that you'll stick with the plan. Of course, there will be times when scheduling surprises or your own lack of motivation will crank up the challenge to keep going. Skipping a day now and then isn't a problem—as long as you don't let one day off turn into three or more. Not only will a longer lapse make it that much harder to get back on track but you'll be postponing the feel-good benefits of working out, as well.

Above all, the key is to make exercise a priority in your life—and to banish the guilt, as well as the excuses, about how much time it takes. Think of exercising as an essential way of taking care of yourself throughout your life, just as regular maintenance, oil changes, and gas fill-ups are essential for your car. If you make time to exercise regularly and find ways to weave it into the tapestry of your life, you're bound to gain a renewed sense of vitality, a verve that can then be channeled toward your family, your work, and other important commitments. Consider it a gift of energy from which everyone in your life will benefit.

## TEN STEALTHY WAYS TO SNEAK IN MORE MOVEMENT

One of the secrets of successfully making movement a regular part of your life is to increase the fun factor. After all, if physical activity is fun or even playfully purposeful, it'll probably feel less like exercise and more like pleasure, which is something we could all use a bit more of in our lives. As an added bonus, you'll wind up burning extra calories with these activities. These lifestyle exercises shouldn't be considered substitutes for formal exercise; they should be viewed as additional ways to fit in more movement throughout the day. What follows are ten pleasant ways to incorporate physical activity into your daily life without even realizing you're doing it:

1. Take the dog for a brisk walk instead of a leisurely stroll.
2. Play tag with your kids instead of watching them play with their friends.
3. Go dancing with your partner instead of to a movie.

4. Play badminton or volleyball instead of sitting on your bottom at a barbecue.
5. Mow the lawn or rake the leaves instead of hiring a neighborhood kid to do it.
6. Take the stairs instead of the elevator at work.
7. Ride bikes to a family picnic instead of driving.
8. Sign up for a charitable walk instead of just writing a check.
9. Spend a rainy afternoon bowling with your kids instead of making cookies.
10. Wash and wax your own car instead of taking it to a drive-through station.

# How to Burn Calories Like a Thin Person

We all know naturally thin, energetic people who can eat whatever their hearts and minds desire—without gaining an ounce. Some researchers have long suspected that these people tend to burn off extra calories because they move more frequently on a daily basis than the rest of us do. Whether they participate in formal exercise or not, these people often move their bodies simply by performing household chores, walking, or fidgeting throughout the day. That's right: fidgeting counts when it comes to burning calories.

In fact, recent research has found that fidgeting is one component of what's called nonexercise activity thermogenesis (NEAT), activities that produce extra body heat and hence burn additional calories in the absence of formal exercise. Best of all, fidgeting, along with other physical activities of daily life such as walking, can actually prevent weight gain when otherwise sedentary, normal-weight adults overeat, allowing them to burn off as much as 69 percent of the additional calories. In a recent study, researchers at the Mayo Clinic in Rochester, Minnesota found that people's energy expenditure—or the rate at which they burned calories—increased when they fidgeted while seated and rose even more when they fidgeted while standing.

The good news is, you can steal the habits of those who fidget naturally in quick, easy ways. Here are seven strategies for burning extra calories:

■ Twirl your hair (if it's long) or the phone cord (if your hair is short) in large circles while you talk on the phone.
■ Use your hand to tap out your favorite tune on the steering wheel while you're driving.

- Pretend you're a ballet dancer and do pliés and relèves while you wash the dishes.
- Set a timer to ring every thirty minutes and stand up and march in place for thirty seconds when it does.
- Sway back and forth, shifting your weight noticeably and rhythmically from one foot to the other while standing in line.
- When sitting with your legs crossed, jiggle whichever foot is on top and periodically uncross and recross your legs.
- When walking, swing your arms as if you were powering yourself along.

## SETTING YOURSELF UP FOR ENERGY-BOOSTING WORKOUTS

Whether you're exercising in an effort to gain better health, more energy, or a slimmer figure, it's wise to do a little preworkout planning to set the stage for success—before swinging into action. This will help you circumvent some of the obstacles that might otherwise hinder your commitment to exercising regularly. Here are some strategies to help you stay moving on the course to increased pep and power.

**CHOOSE ACTIVITIES YOU REALLY ENJOY:** If exercise feels like a chore, you'll be less likely to stick with it over the long haul. If you tend to like group activities, consider joining a local soccer, softball, or rowing team—or sign up for an aerobics class at the gym. If you prefer to exercise with a friend, cultivate an exercise buddy who enjoys the same activities you do and is someone whose company you enjoy.

**FIND WAYS TO FIT EXERCISE INTO YOUR LIFE:** If free time is a precious commodity and you're hard pressed to fit in regular workouts, be creative: instead of meeting a friend for lunch, make a date to go for a hike; instead of hanging out with your kids after school, take them for a bike ride or in-line skating. Of course, you should pick a time of day and a setting that makes sense for you. If it's easier for you to stick with a morning workout before the day's events interfere with your best-laid plans, set your alarm and get moving as the sun comes up. But if you enjoy working out after work because it helps you relieve stress, try to plan your day accordingly.

**GIVE YOURSELF AN ATTITUDE ADJUSTMENT:** Instead of thinking of exercise as something you *should* do, start viewing it as something you *want* to do because it's a gift to yourself—a gift of stamina, strength, and stress relief. This way, you'll look forward to working out and you'll focus on the enjoyable aspects of exercise.

**SET SPECIFIC, MEASURABLE GOALS:** There's no better way to feel the payoff for all your hard workouts than to realize that you're actually achieving something. The key to setting goals is to make them concrete, realistic, and action-oriented: "I'm going to start exercising for thirty minutes four times per week" rather than "I'm going to get fit." This way, your goal will spell out exactly what you need to do to attain it. If you then keep an exercise diary that tracks your progress over time, you'll have a built-in incentive to keep going—because you'll see that you're on a winning course.

**OFFER YOURSELF VARIETY IN THE SPORTING LIFE:** To stave off boredom, burnout, and overuse injuries, it's important to vary your routine with cross-training (biking one day, walking the next) and a change of scenery (hitting alternate trails on occasion). This can help prevent injuries that result from placing too much stress and strain on the same muscles, bones, and joints day after day—and will help keep your exercise life interesting.

**WEAR THE RIGHT SHOES:** That means well-constructed sport-specific shoes (running shoes for running, tennis shoes for tennis, walking shoes for walking, and so on) that offer plenty of cushioning and support where you need it most. This will help minimize the impact on your feet and, hence, the rest of your body. If you need to invest in a pair of new shoes, shop at a store that specializes in athletic footwear (it's more likely to have a large inventory) and go late in the day, when your feet are most swollen.

**DRESS FOR THE OCCASION:** In hot weather, wear light-colored, loose-fighting clothes in a lightweight fabric that allows sweat to evaporate. Natural fabrics such as cotton allow the skin to breathe and the heat to escape from your body; synthetic fabrics such as polyester and Lycra don't. It's also a good idea to wear a cotton baseball cap or visor to keep the sun off your face. In cold temperatures, wear layers of clothing so that you can peel them off as your body temperature climbs during exercise and put them back on when you finish your workout; again, it's smart to wear a hat, in this instance to avoid losing heat through the top of your head.

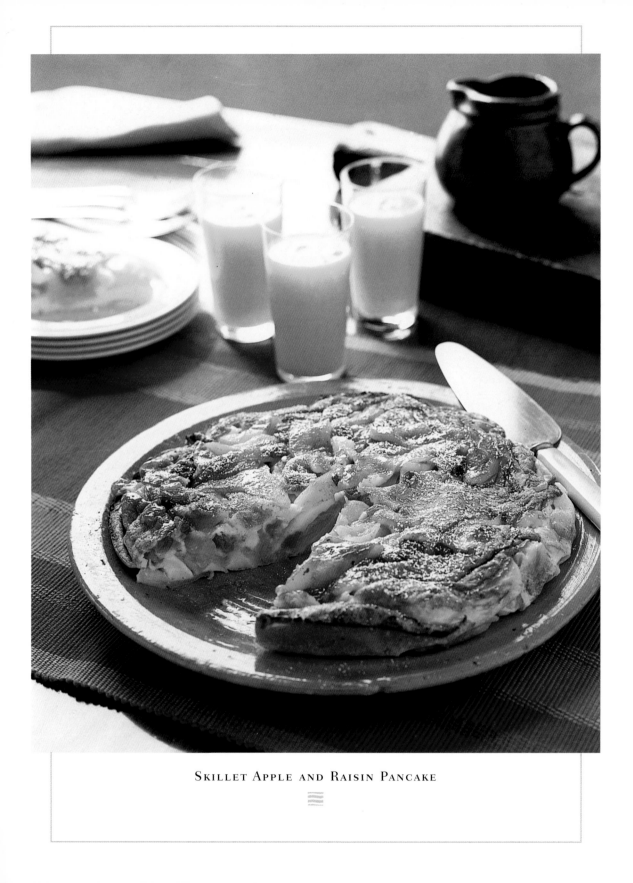

SKILLET APPLE AND RAISIN PANCAKE

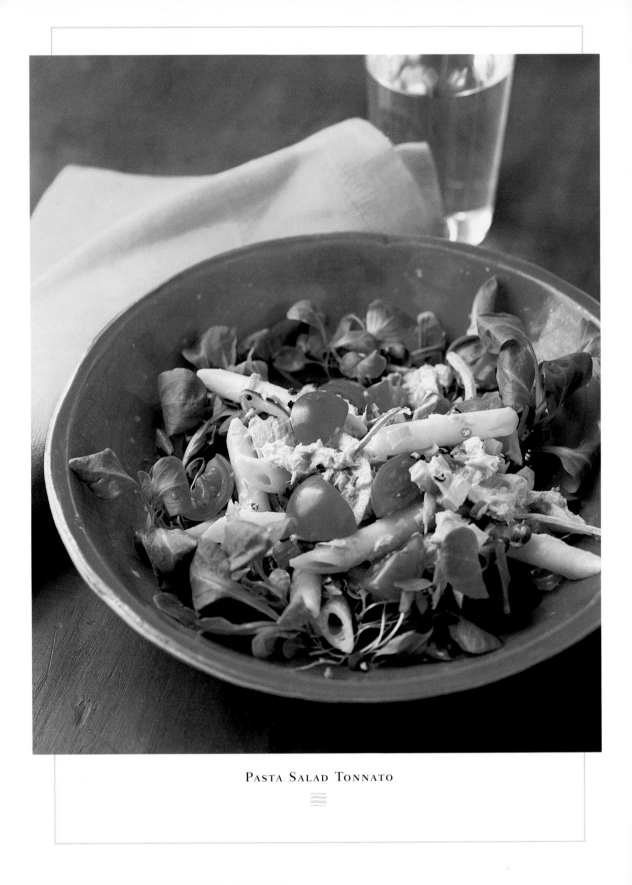

PASTA SALAD TONNATO

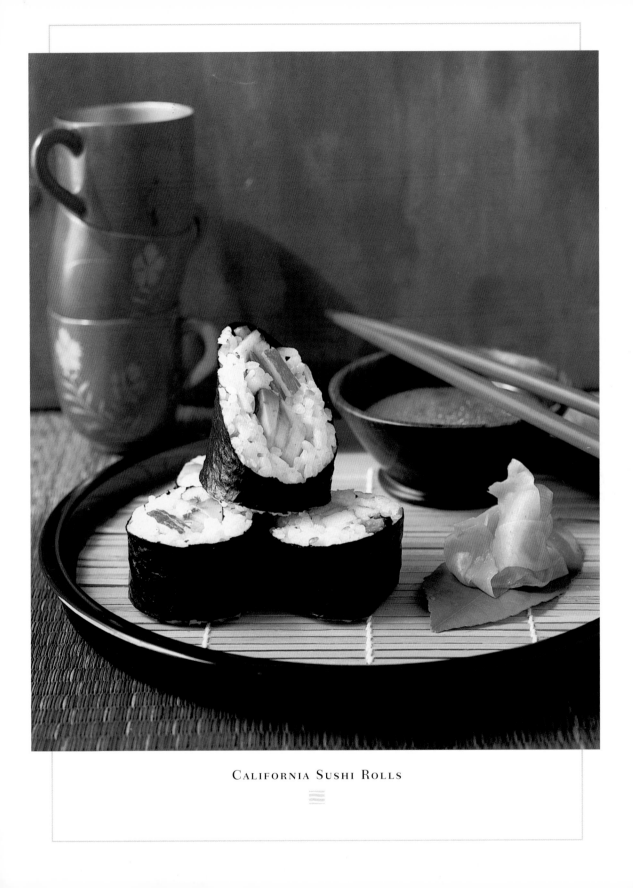

CALIFORNIA SUSHI ROLLS

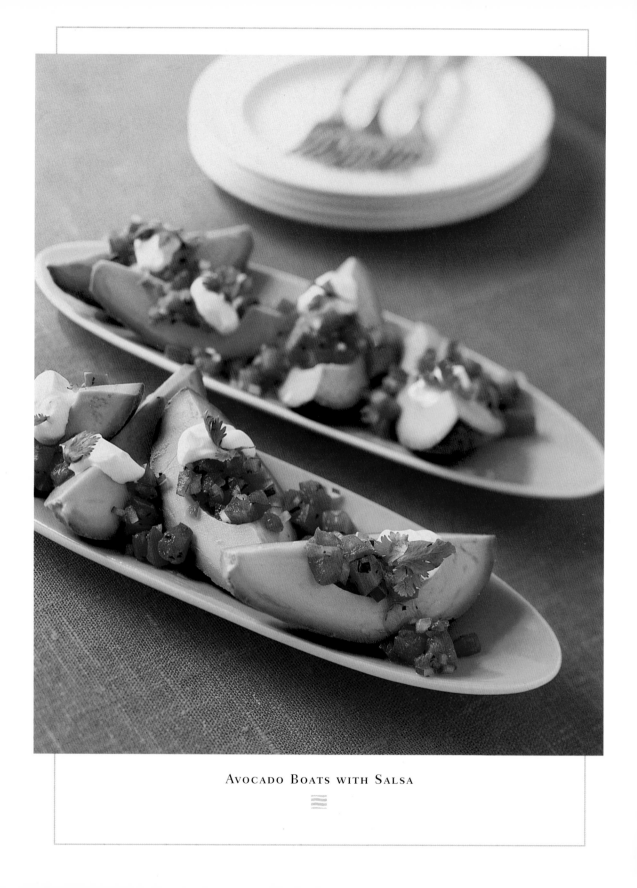

AVOCADO BOATS WITH SALSA

When it comes to making exercise a habit, attitude is more than half the battle. Do you have the right mind-set to get moving and stay moving? Or is your mind-set holding you back before you even get started? To find out, answer the following questions Yes or No.

1. Does the very idea of exercising bore you?
2. Are you a pro at finding excuses not to engage in physical activities?
3. If a friend invited you to go on a bike ride, would you suggest meeting for lunch instead?
4. Do you get tired just watching someone else work out?
5. Do you choose the elevator over the stairs every chance you get?
6. Have you given up on exercising because you weren't satisfied with the results you obtained in the past?
7. Are you waiting until you lose weight to start exercising?
8. Do you hate the idea of breaking a sweat?
9. Do you resolve to take up exercise year after year but never seem to get around to doing it?
10. Do you often choose to drive on errands that you could walk to?

Now give yourself one point for each time you answered Yes. If you scored:

**6–10 points: You're on the wrong side of the starting gate.** First of all, you're full of excuses for shirking workouts, but you're only cheating yourself—of a natural way to lose weight, boost your mood, and decrease your risks of cancer, heart disease, and diabetes, among other chronic health conditions. Your best bet is to make an honest list of what's really holding you back, along with the pros and cons of starting to exercise; then decide how to counter each reason for not exercising with a possible solution. For example, if you're not making the time to exercise because you'd feel uncomfortable having other people see you work out, you might consider walking on your own or doing an exercise video in the privacy of your home.

**3–5 points: You're facing a few hurdles along the fitness path.** Whether you're truly sedentary or you just have a few obstacles to overcome in becoming proexercise, you'd be wise to give your excuses a reality check, then set goals that you can tackle one by one. If you've been unhappy with the results of previous exercise efforts, for example, maybe you expected too much too soon. While exercise can begin to feel good in a matter of days, it takes most people about a month to see real cardiovascular and strength benefits. In the meantime, it helps to give yourself as much positive feedback as possible: keep a graph that shows the length and frequency of your workouts and you'll get automatic encouragement to keep the positive trend going; plus, if you notice how much easier your workouts become over time, that's an added incentive to keep up the good work.

0–2 points: You're ready to reap the energy-boosting benefits of exercise. When it comes right down to it, you're actually proexercise. You just may not have thought of yourself that way. But there may be one or two challenges that are keeping you from wholeheartedly embracing the active life. Maybe the will is there but you haven't found the most enjoyable way(s) for you to exercise. Or maybe you've simply overlooked golden opportunities to sneak in more movement on a regular basis. Open your eyes! Start looking for new opportunities to fit in short or social bouts of exercise and be willing to try new physical activities. Not only are you likely to discover the energizing effects of exercise, but becoming more physical can actually become a catalyst that prompts you to take better care of yourself in other ways, too.

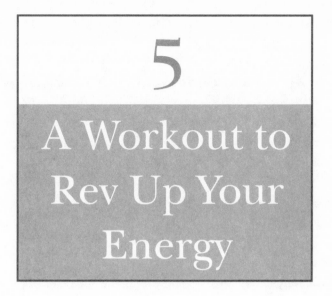

# 5

## A Workout to Rev Up Your Energy

When I was overweight, there was no balance in my life. I saw things as black or white, wonderful or terrible, exhilarating or terrifying. I'm passionate by nature, but seeing the world in such extremes made every day like a ride on a roller coaster. Of course my body was tired because I rarely gave it what it needed to be energetic. I routinely skipped meals, thinking I could afford to miss the calories, and some of the fad diets I tried so limited my intake of nutrients that it was all I could do to get up in the morning. I exercised sporadically.

In my haste to become thin I used to focus so much on the start and finish of my diet that I ignored the best part of the journey, which is in between. You can't hurry change, and it takes patience to stay motivated as you reach for a far-off goal. There are still days when I just want to throw up my hands and declare an end to dieting and exercise. Deep down I never mean it, of course, but at times like these it helps me to look to others who inspire me.

People who run marathons amaze me. Finishing a twenty-six-mile race is an extraordinary feat by any measure, yet I've known Weight Watchers members who have became marathoners. One member, Beth, started walking after she shed nearly 100 pounds. In time she progressed to jogging and then running, gradually increasing her strength and endurance. Sure, Beth was an unlikely marathoner at first, but now she's a veteran, having run many of them. There are plenty of people like Beth who achieve vitality beyond their expectations once they get into fitness. Whether you like to walk, run, lift weights, swim, or dance, just settle into a fitness routine you really enjoy, and there's no telling how far you can go.

I'm here to say that what you've heard about the mood-enhancing benefits of eating right and exercising are true. In becoming more physically active, my outlook definitely improved, I had better concentration, and I certainly had more stamina. Seeing a firmer figure emerge was gratifying, too, but more important, it gave me a greater feeling of power over my body and mind that I'd not felt in quite a long time. Of course, being active has to go hand in hand with learning to eat better. With both, I find the anger and frustration I'd felt with myself about my weight was replaced with patience and even compassion. I had never really understood how certain situations and feelings would trigger my destructive habits. Now, knowing my triggers has helped me get to the root of—and remedy—my weight problem.

Working out with Josh, as well as the discipline of tracking meals and making good food choices, made me the driver of my own life—and this felt really good. If eating out of anger was self-destructive, then heading off a binge and sticking to healthy meals and exercising are more positive alternatives.

Yet traveling as much as I do makes it tough for me to keep up my fitness routine. So I've accepted the fact that there will be times, sometime entire weeks, when it's impractical or impossible for me to exercise. I don't dwell on what I've missed. Rather, I stay committed to getting back on track with my routine as soon as I'm back home. I listen to my body because it will tell me how hard I should push my-

## Time Out, Please

"Though I'm able to work full throttle on most days, I draw the line when I'm on vacation. There will always be reasons to stay in touch with the office, but with advance planning and clear guidelines on calls and faxes, you can make a great escape. When I'm on holiday, I may speak with my office once each week. I insist on staying busy doing things that I, and my family, enjoy."

self, but it's never a question of whether or not I feel up to working out. I think the Nike slogan sums it up best: "Just do it."

And my healthier attitude about working out has spilled into my thinking about eating right. None of us is born with an innate sense of good nutrition. We learn our eating habits and preferences from an early age, and short of studying nutrition in school, most of us bungle through life eating a hodgepodge of foods we like and meals we think are healthy. Americans especially seem to equate large, hearty portions with health, but in fact overeating is one of the worst things you can do. Since joining Weight Watchers, I've become fascinated by the food myths that are still rampant. What we grew up believing may have no basis in fact. For example, I was raised on a farm in the English countryside, where a hearty breakfast was necessary if you were facing a day of heavy manual labor. It's true that a meal of eggs with grilled sausages with a stack of toast with full-fat butter could stoke the furnace of a busy farmhand. But unless you are going to be very physically active, starting off the day with a high-fat meal may leave you feeling lethargic rather than energized.

I've realized that it's knowing all these little bits of nutrition and fitness information that has helped me live a more full, energetic life. Somewhere along the way, I consciously or unconsciously realized that I had to learn such things in order to change my life—for the better. By virtue of the fact that you are reading this book, you are taking a step toward making changes in your life in ways that will ultimately give you more energy. If feeling out of control leaves you feeling exasperated, learning to take control will energize you. Consider the analogy of two pregnant women in labor: one of the women is distraught and powerless with each contraction while the other uses Lamaze techniques to systematically work through the discomfort. Both women are in pain, but they could not be more different in their sense of control over the situation. I urge you to read this chapter carefully and do the exercises, which will help you regain more control over your feelings and how you live your life.

# Use It or Lose It

The old saying "Use it or lose it" could just as easily apply to energy as to body strength and fitness. In addition to all the physiological benefits that are associated with regular exercise—improved breathing and circulation, a more efficient metabolism, enhanced immune function, and so on—movement can also simply make you feel vibrant and invigorated. It makes you feel robust, healthy, and alive. Being sedentary, on the other hand, can make you feel sluggish and sleepy because when you sit or lie still for long periods of time, many of your body's functions—including your circulation—slow down. This is a more immediate effect of a sedentary life, compared to the long-term effects of increasing your risks of all kinds of illnesses and ailments.

Once you resolve to get moving and actually launch your plan of action, you'll soon discover how exercise can pump up your energy level, both physically and psychologically. In all likelihood, you'll begin to feel more vigorous in body and more buoyant in mind and spirit within a matter of weeks. These positive feelings can become addictive and can even fuel a commitment to being more physically active. Not only can this lifestyle change make you feel more energetic, but it can help you take other steps to improve your health and manage your weight, as well. And when you begin to lose body fat and gain muscle definition, these changes in your physical appearance can give you a self-confidence boost that can also be energizing.

But if you truly want to reap the maximum energy-enhancing effects of exercise, you'll need to pay attention to your approach. After all, the right exercise regimen can jump-start your energy, while the wrong one can squander it. This is why it's important to heed exercise Rule Number One: Choose activities that you enjoy. It's hardly surprising that there are different strokes for different folks when it comes to exercise. Try to ignore or deny this truism, and you could wind up sabotaging your efforts to get physical. After all, if you don't enjoy your workouts, you'll be less likely to stick with them or treat them as sacred in the midst of a perpetually time-strapped schedule and more likely to experience boredom or burnout. The bottom line: if you don't find a way to enjoy your workouts, you'll be more likely to become an exercise dropout. On the other hand, if you can discover physical activities or sports that bring you pleasure and make you feel good, you'll probably make them a priority in your life and look forward to them.

# Exercising Your Options

The only way to discover physical activities you truly enjoy is through trial and error. In the United States, the most commonly chosen form of exercise is walking, according to research by the Centers for Disease Control and Prevention. This is followed by gardening or yard work, stretching exercises, riding a bike or exercise bike, weight lifting (or other strengthening exercises), stair climbing, jogging or running, aerobics or aerobic dance, swimming, and playing basketball.

Luckily, there are plenty of choices when it comes to exercise, and the key to making it a habit for life is to discover what's fun for you and what works for you. But rather than stick solely with one form of activity, you also may want to venture beyond what's familiar. You might want to broaden your repertoire of activities by adding new ones that are in sync with your personality, goals, and lifestyle. If you crave the camaraderie and spirit of a group experience, you might consider joining a local softball, volleyball, or soccer team, for example. If the hours you spend exercising are the only ones you have to be alone with your thoughts and this is something you treasure, walking, jogging, swimming, bike riding, or in-line skating may appeal to you. If you thrive on competition, you might take up tennis, squash, or basketball. If you tend to feel energized by spending time in nature, consider hiking, mountain biking, kayaking, or rowing—or cross-country skiing or snowshoeing during the winter months. On the other hand, if you feel invigorated after pushing your limits against machines, you might prefer to alternate among the treadmill, stair climber, stationary bike, cross-country ski machine, elliptical trainer, or rowing machine at the gym.

When choosing activities, you also may want to consider what type of energy you're trying to cultivate. If what you crave is calm but invigorating energy, you might do well with gentler forms of movement such as yoga, tai chi, chi gong, or Pilates. But if what you want is a high-octane workout that will leave you feeling revved up, high-intensity aerobic dance, kickboxing, Tae Bo, or Spinning may give you the high-charged sensation you desire. But again, different forms of exercise affect people differently, so experiment to see what gives you the workout intensity you want and the type of energy you crave.

# Avoiding Exercise Mistakes

While there's no question that a well-crafted exercise plan can fuel your energy, unhealthy approaches to working out can actually leave you feeling drained. This is partly because there's an optimal zone in terms of intensity, duration, and frequency of exercise. But it can be easy to cross the line into under- or overdoing it. Here are five mistakes to sidestep so that they don't sideline you:

**MISTAKE 1: *Getting Overly Gung Ho About Exercise***

At first blush, it may seem like a good idea to work out vigorously every day if you're trying to get fit, but in fact not if it's robbing you of energy. This is an especially common problem among beginning exercisers and people who were in shape at one time and want to get back into shape quickly. The truth is, your body needs some rest between workouts and time to replenish energy stores and repair muscles and connective tissue. This is why experts often recommend at least one day of rest per week if you exercise vigorously aerobically. This is also why it's important to avoid strength training on consecutive days since muscles need ample time to recover from the stress you're placing on them.

Once you've begun exercising somewhat regularly, you can use soreness as a way to figure out if you deserve a break today. If you feel anything greater than slight soreness or if you feel just plain exhausted the morning after you've exercised vigorously, either exercise lightly that day or take the day off. Or, you could get into the habit of working out every other day; just don't take off more than two days in a row because you could fall out of the exercise habit altogether.

**MISTAKE 2: *Intensifying Your Workouts Too Quickly***

When you get hooked on exercise, it's easy to let your enthusiasm and ambition take over, but sometimes these positive attributes can push the envelope too far. After all, just as it isn't prudent to switch from exercising every time there's a full moon to exercising every day, you shouldn't suddenly double the length of your regular run—from thirty minutes to sixty minutes, for instance—without working up to it gradually. These sorts of zealous jumps in intensity could zap your energy, give you an overuse injury, or make you sick. What's more, recent research from the University of Alberta in Edmonton, Canada, found that when people who weren't in shape overexercised, they experienced emotional distress afterward.

Other signs of overtraining include decreased performance, loss of coordination, an elevated heart rate in the morning, frequent headaches, loss of appetite, gastrointestinal disturbances, decreased resistance to infection, and unusual muscle soreness. A good rule of thumb for avoiding the perils of overdoing it when starting a program: don't increase the length or intensity of your workouts by more than 25 percent per week.

**MISTAKE 3:** *Exercising When You Haven't Had Anything to Eat for Hours*
No, you shouldn't exercise on a full stomach. But neither is it smart to work out when you're running on empty because this is like setting off on a long road trip with an empty tank of gas. To prevent your energy from fizzling out halfway through a workout, have a carbohydrate-rich snack with a little protein—¼ cup of trail mix or a few whole-wheat crackers smeared lightly with peanut butter, for example—at least an hour before exercising. Also, make sure you start your exercise session well hydrated: Drink 8 to 16 ounces of water or another noncaffeinated fluid thirty to sixty minutes before your workout. And it is certainly advisable to consume fluids regularly throughout your workout.

**MISTAKE 4:** *Expecting to Be Able to Do a New Activity*
*for the Same Duration as a More Familiar One*
When you first take up swimming or rowing, for example, it's simply unrealistic to expect your workout to last as long as your habitual jog in the neighborhood. After all, your skill may not be up to par, and you'll be using different muscles, which may not be well conditioned and may not have stamina. So it's almost like starting from ground zero. That's why it's wise to test the waters by starting slowly instead of trying to do too much too soon. You might swim for twenty minutes your first time out—taking rest breaks as needed—then see how you feel the next day before adding to your time. And take the talk test occasionally while you're rowing: you should feel as though you're getting exercise, but you shouldn't be huffing and puffing; you should be able to talk but not sing. If you're too out of breath to talk, you should slow down the pace.

**MISTAKE 5:** *Succumbing to the "I'm Too Tired to Exercise" Excuse*
There's no question: it can be difficult to drag yourself to the gym when you're feeling beat from head to toe. But if you shirk your workout, you'll never know whether exercise would have energized you. A better strategy: stick with the ten-minute rule. Force yourself to go out and exercise for at least ten minutes. If at that point you still feel exhausted, give yourself permission to stop. But in all likelihood, exercise will help you feel better and you'll choose to keep going.

# MOBILIZING CHI

The whole notion of awakening your personal energy has a different twist in Eastern teachings. There, it's not about simply gaining more get-up-and-go but about enhancing the flow of internal or life energy that naturally courses through our minds and bodies. Different cultures espouse similar beliefs about a vital energy on which people can draw for physical, emotional, and spiritual well-being. In Chinese traditions, it's called *qi* (or *chi*); in Japan, it's known as *ki;* in India, *prana.* By any name, it's considered the stuff of life, the life force that pulses through every body.

It is a concept that's somewhat foreign to Western cultures—and there isn't a word in the English language that captures its essence precisely. "If you want to think of Qi as the energy that creates and animates material and spiritual being, the life force, or the breath of life, you will come close to understanding Qi," notes Misha Ruth Cohen, a Doctor of Oriental Medicine and author of *The Chinese Way to Healing: Many Paths to Wholeness* (Perigee). The thinking is that when this vital energy flows freely and smoothly, the body's organs and systems are in a state of harmony; when it doesn't, illness and fatigue can occur. Taking steps to fine-tune and unblock clogged energy channels in your body is believed to result in greater well-being, improved health, and relief from everyday ailments such as back pain, menstrual cramps, digestive distress, and other nagging symptoms.

There are many ways to stimulate the flow of energy; some are more active than others. Among the disciplines that use movement to mobilize your inner energy are:

QI GONG: An ancient healing technique, qi gong is the basic exercise system within Chinese medicine, and it's a bit like moving meditation. By combining stretches, rhythmic breathing exercises, visualization, and circular, flowing movements, the aim is to change the flow of energy inside and outside the body. Practitioners believe that doing this can have a positive effect on health, physical performance, and emotional well-being, as well as slowing the aging process.

TAI CHI: Though it is best known as a martial art, tai chi incorporates slow, fluid movements that are based on forces in nature. These movements are believed to open the body's energy gates, allowing the *chi* from nature and the universe to enter the body's pathways and harmonize the circulation of *chi* within the body. Its proponents say this reduces stress, promotes relaxation, and enhances balance, strength, and physical control.

**YOGA:** Not only does the ancient Indian art of yoga enhance flexibility and balance, but it relies on gentle stretches, precise poses, and specific breathing patterns to increase energy. The goal is to open the body's energy channels and create different effects—such as fiery energy; sleepier, more inert energy; or pure, illuminating energy—with different poses and breathing patterns. Performed properly, its proponents maintain that yoga can reduce stress and fatigue, improve coordination and body awareness, and enhance general well-being.

Another way to enhance the flow of internal energy is with bodywork techniques. Here, the idea is to apply external sources of energy or to use external manipulation to boost and balance an individual's own depleted energy. With these techniques, you concentrate on relaxing your body and mind, while expert hands (and sometimes feet and elbows) do the work of cultivating *chi.* The following techniques can be used on their own or as supplements to the moving disciplines.

**ACUPUNCTURE:** Based on the idea that there are energy channels or meridians running through the body, acupuncture is believed to stimulate or adjust the flow of the body's internal energy through the placement of hair-thin needles in designated points along major meridians that are spread symmetrically throughout the body. The exact placement of the needles depends on what's being treated, but the idea is that by unblocking the flow of energy, fatigue will be relieved, as will a variety of symptoms, such as pain, inflammation, and tension. Advocates also believe that acupuncture can be used to prevent illness by fine-tuning the flow of *chi* through these channels and thwarting imbalances.

**ACUPRESSURE:** This technique is often thought of as a specialized form of massage, but it's based on the same principles as acupuncture. Acupressurists apply pressure to key points along the same meridians with their fingers, hands, elbows, or feet. The goal is to stimulate circulation, induce relaxation, and reestablish or redirect the flow of *chi,* thereby promoting healing and returning the body to a state of harmony.

**REFLEXOLOGY:** In this form of foot therapy, reflexology practitioners believe there are key energy zones in the body that correspond to specific areas of the feet. The idea is that when these zones are manipulated by a practitioner's hands (or even a special stick), the body's energy can be brought back into balance and health can be improved.

**REIKI:** The name comes from the Japanese words *rei* (which means "spirit") and *ki* (which means "energy"), and the practice is believed to reduce stress as well as relieving headaches, stomach trouble, muscle spasms, and other forms of discomfort. This hands-on approach uses the power of a practitioner's touch to influence the flow of energy into injured areas and throughout the body. Rather than manipulating muscles, ligaments, or other body tissues, a reiki practitioner simply lays his or her hands on the client in particular patterns that facilitate the flow of energy from the practitioner into the client's body.

**SHIATSU:** Developed in Japan, this technique is a type of massage that involves vigorous, rhythmic pressing of acupressure points for brief periods of time. The practitioner applies pressure along key points of the body using his or her fingers, elbows, even feet—similar to the way in which an acupuncturist would apply needles—to unclog blocked energy channels and ease tension and fatigue. Shiatsu is supposed to be especially beneficial for back problems, neck and shoulder pain, even headaches and digestive problems.

## Walking: Your Basic Energy Fitness Plan

When it comes to fitness activities, one of the biggest advantages of walking is that you already know how to do it. You just put one foot in front of the other, and you're on your way. Plus, walking doesn't require a lot of fancy gear. All you have to do is put on your shoes and head out the door. Besides, it's an ideal form of exercise for several reasons: not only can it help you slim down, but it offers all sorts of surprising health benefits—from enhancing your immune function and protecting against bone loss to lowering your cholesterol and blood pressure to boosting your mood. It's also a relatively low-impact form of exercise, which means it won't put too much wear and tear on your joints.

You can use walking as the foundation of a complete fitness plan—if you include stretching exercises during your warm-up and cool-down periods (think of these as bookends to your workout) and break up your bouts of walking with resistance training in the form of calisthenics. This adds up to an interval-circuit program that will enhance your aerobic capacity, muscle strength, and flexibility, which will work together to boost your energy level and your overall fitness.

Before beginning this or any exercise program, it's a good idea to get clearance from your health care provider, just in case you have a medical condition that may limit your activity. Once you get the green light, you'll be ready to roll. You should strive to do the following walking program at least five days per week. If you've been completely sedentary until now, you may want to start by doing it at least three days the first week and up to five days by the third week. If your muscles feel sore twenty-four to forty-eight after doing this, don't worry; this is actually a normal physiological response to starting an exercise program that uses muscles in a manner they're unaccustomed to. The phenomenon is called "delayed onset muscle soreness" (DOMS), and it's the result of tiny tears in the muscle fibers. This will go away in a day or two; a warm bath and massaging the sore muscles can help in the meantime.

## HOW TO STRIDE RIGHT

Before you get started on this or any other walking program, you'll want to make sure you're walking the right way. Yes, you were born to do the locomotion, but form counts if you want to maximize the fitness benefits and minimize the potential for injury. Here's how to make sure you're striding right:

**POSTURE:** Keep your spine in its proper alignment by standing tall from head to toe. Keep your shoulders relaxed and down, your chest up, your abdominal muscles pulled in, and your chin parallel to the ground. As you walk, keep your eyes focused on where you're going straight ahead, not on the ground.

**ARMS:** Relax your arms and bend them at the elbows. As you step out with one foot, swing the opposite arm forward, then back, as the other arm and foot come forward. Be sure to keep your elbows close to your side and your hands in a relaxed fist (imagine holding an egg). Your hands should never rise higher than chest level.

**FEET:** With each step, you'll land on your heel, with your toes pointing toward the sky, and roll through the foot, pushing off from the toes. Stick with a stride length that feels natural and a pace that feels comfortable. You can always increase either element once you get going.

Before each exercise session, you'll want to warm up your cardiovascular system and your muscles by walking at a comfortable pace for two to three minutes. (Keep in mind: You'll need a sports watch for this workout since you'll be timing your intervals.) Then spend two to three minutes doing gentle calisthenics such as jumping jacks, progressively larger arm circles, and the following stretches. Remember: the goal with these exercises is to limber up and loosen up your muscles before walking.

To loosen up your calf muscles, stand a few feet away from a wall and lean forward, placing both hands against the wall for support. Bring your right leg forward, bending your knee and placing your foot flat on the ground. Lean toward the wall until you feel a good stretch in your left calf muscle. Hold this position for five seconds. Repeat with the other leg.

To stretch the quadriceps (the muscle along the front of your thigh), stand on the floor and put your weight on your right foot. Bend your left knee, and with your left hand pull the left heel straight back toward your buttocks. Hold for five seconds. Switch legs and repeat.

## Week One

Once you've spent five minutes limbering up, start walking at a moderately brisk pace (no more strenuous than what you would rate as feeling "somewhat hard") for five minutes, then hit the deck and spend two minutes doing **abdominal crunches:** Lie on your back with your knees bent, your feet flat on the floor hip width apart, chin tucked to chest, and lace your fingers behind your head, without straining your neck. Tilt your pelvis toward the ceiling, press your lower back into the floor, and try to lift your shoulder blades off the floor without pulling on your neck. Hold this position for a count, then lower your shoulder blades back to the floor. If you can't do crunches continuously for two minutes, take a brief rest, then do more.

When your two minutes are up, get back on your feet and step lively as you walk for five minutes. Then hit the floor and do **modified push-ups** for two minutes: Get down on the floor on your hands and knees (making sure that your hands are directly below your shoulders), and cross your ankles so that your feet are off the ground. Bend your elbows and slowly lower yourself toward the floor as far as you can comfortably go, then push yourself straight up from the floor. Do as many as you can in two minutes, even if you need to rest for a few moments.

Next, set off walking briskly for another five minutes, then spend the next two minutes doing **lunges:** Stand with your feet hip width apart and place your hands on your hips. Take a large step forward with your right foot, bending both knees. Keep your back straight and your chin parallel to the ground, and sink down until your right hamstring is parallel to the floor. While contracting your abdominal muscles, push back with the right foot to the starting position. Repeat with the left leg and continue doing repetitions on each side.

Now it's time to cool down. After each exercise session, you'll want to walk slowly for two minutes instead of stopping cold, then spend several minutes stretching. This time, the focus of stretching will be on enhancing flexibility since the muscles are now truly warm and pliable. This will help you improve your range of motion for various muscle groups and joints. (See "The Cool-Down Protocol" on page 96.)

**Your total workout time** (including warm-up and cool-down): 31 minutes

## Week Two

After warming up and loosening up, walk at a moderately brisk pace for seven minutes. Then hit the floor and spend two minutes doing abdominal crunches. Return to walking again for seven minutes, then do modified push-ups for two minutes. Next spend seven minutes walking, then do lunges for two minutes. After that, you're ready to spend some time cooling down and working on flexibility before getting on with your day.

**Your total workout time** (including warm-up and cool-down): 37 minutes

## Week Three

Spend five minutes doing your warm-up and stretching routine. Then walk at a moderately brisk pace for nine minutes. This time, you're going to take a three-minute interval for the strengthening exercises and divide it evenly among crunches, modified push-ups, and lunges, spending one minute on each. After that, resume walking for another nine minutes, then repeat the muscle strengthening routine, again alternating between the three exercises. Do one final walking tour (for nine minutes), followed by the strengthening exercises. Spend five minutes cooling down; then you're ready to call it quits.

**Your total workout time** (including warm-up and cool-down): 46 minutes

## Week Four

After the usual five-minute warm-up and stretching period, you'll be walking for twelve-minute stints this week. These will be interspersed with three four-minute sessions of strengthening moves—with one minute each for crunches, modified push-ups, lunges, and half squats. To do **half-squats:** Stand with your knees shoulder width apart and your hands extended in front of you for balance. Keep your head up and back straight, bend your knees and slowly push your butt down and out as if you were going to sit on a chair (but don't bend your knees beyond a 90-degree angle), then slowly raise yourself up again.

**Your total workout time** (including warm-up and cool-down): 58 minutes

Chances are, you'll end up walking at a faster pace over the four weeks as your fitness level improves. What you'll want to do is maintain a pace that feels somewhat hard, based on your own rating of perceived exertion. This way you'll continuously improve your level of conditioning, and, by gradually extending the duration of your workouts, you'll be improving the calorie-burning effects, too.

# THE COOL-DOWN PROTOCOL

At the end of a workout, many people simply call it quits and head to the shower. By doing this, they're shortchanging themselves of a prime opportunity to help their bodies recover from exercise and enhance their flexibility. The idea behind a cool-down is to spend a few additional minutes easing out of exercise—by walking at a gentle pace, for example—then to take advantage of the warmth and pliability of your muscles by doing some serious stretching. Here are seven exercises that will improve the range of motion for various joints and muscles throughout your body:

**TO IMPROVE THE FLEXIBILITY OF YOUR CALF MUSCLES:** Stand on a step with one foot squarely on the step, the other with the ball of the foot on the step and the heel hanging off. Hold on to a wall or railing for balance, and gently press the heel down off the step. Hold for twenty to thirty seconds. Repeat with the other foot.

**TO STRETCH THE QUADRICEPS:** Stand on the floor and put your weight on your right foot. Bend your left knee and with your left hand, pull the left heel straight back toward your buttocks. Hold for twenty to thirty seconds. Switch legs and repeat.

**TO STRETCH THE HAMSTRINGS** (the muscles along the back of your thigh): Lie flat on your back with both legs straight. Grasp your left leg behind the thigh and pull it in to your chest. Hold this position, then extend your left leg toward the ceiling. Hold this position, then bring your left knee back to your chest and pull your toes over toward your shin with your left hand. Stretch the back of the leg by attempting to straighten your knee. Repeat for the other leg.

**TO STRETCH YOUR LOWER BACK:** Kneel on all fours on the floor with your hands shoulder width apart, and round your back and shoulders as if you were a mad cat that's ready to pounce, exhaling and tightening your abdominal muscles as you do so. Hold for five to ten seconds, then relax your muscles and release your back into its natural curve. Do this four to five times.

Then lie on the floor with your knees bent and gently tilt your pelvis so that your back is flat on the floor. Pull your right knee to your chest, while the left stays extended along the floor, and hold it for fifteen seconds. Switch legs. Then pull both knees to your chest and hug them there for thirty seconds.

**TO STRETCH YOUR CHEST:** Stand up and bring both elbows up and out to the side almost like wings, while keeping your hands in front of your chest. Try to squeeze your shoulder blades together behind you. Hold for fifteen seconds.

**TO IMPROVE SHOULDER FLEXIBILITY:** Extend your left arm in front of you at chest level. Grab your left arm at the elbow joint with your right hand and gently pull your arm across your chest until you feel a good stretch in your shoulder. Switch sides and repeat.

# Jazzing Up Your Walking Workout

Once this walking program begins to feel like a stroll in the park, you can spice it up or pump it up in various ways. Not only will this ensure that your workouts stay interesting and challenging, but it will increase the calorie-burning effects as well. After all, the more fit you become, the more it will take to push your pulse rate high enough so that you are truly working in your aerobic target zone. This is because your heart and lungs will be able to function much more efficiently (your energy reserve will be higher), which means you'll have to exercise harder to achieve the same benefits. Here are four ways to maximize the calorie-burning effects and aerobic requirements of any walking program.

### Bring Your Arms into the Picture

Feel as though you're neglecting your upper body with your walking routine? You don't have to. You can pump your arms in an exaggerated fashion to get your upper body involved. Or you can use products such as an oversize belt with retractable cords that provide resistance as you pull them or poles that you place strategically to propel yourself along. Neither will build much arm strength—you need to do strength-training exercises for that—but they can help tone and shape your muscles, especially if you've been sedentary. And these gadgets can boost the calorie-burning effect: a study at the University of Wisconsin–La Crosse found that when people used specially designed poles while walking, they burned 22 percent more calories and increased the aerobic intensity of their workout by 23 percent.

### Add Gentle Speed Play

The idea behind this strategy is to periodically add bursts of speed so that you burn calories faster and increase your heart rate. Here's how it works: After warming up by walking at a comfortable pace and stretching, hit the trail and stride at a reasonable pace, maintaining proper form, for three minutes. Then pick up the pace for the next two minutes. Back down to an easier speed for three minutes, then walk even faster than before for the next three minutes. Continue alternating the pace of your walking for the duration of your workout. This technique is called interval training, and it burns calories and increases your level of conditioning faster than walking at a steady pace. It also gets you out of your comfort zone and mixes up the workout, making it more interesting and challenging. And it can even give you an invigorating confidence boost—by making you realize that you can walk faster than you thought you could.

## Become a Fast Walker

If you reach a point where you feel as though you've maxed out on the fitness benefits of walking, here's a great solution: Fast walking. It'll pump up the calorie-burning benefits—and the cardiovascular effects, to boot.

How to do it: Stand tall with your spine in its proper alignment—your sternum lifted, your shoulders down and pulled back, your chin parallel to the ground. You'll be planting your feet similarly to regular fitness walking—heel first with your toes pulled up hard, then rolling through the foot and pushing off the ball of your foot. But this time you'll be placing your feet one in front of the other (in a straight line), almost as if you were walking on a tightrope. Also, the motion of your hips will be slightly different from that of regular walking: as you place your front foot on the ground with your weight on the rear foot, your rear hip will sink down and rock out to the side; as you shift your weight to the front foot, you'll let the front hip roll to the side, then you'll lift your rear foot and plant it in front. It may sound tricky, but it's actually a very smooth, fluid action, a bit like making a sideways figure eight with your hips.

One of the keys to fast walking is to pump your arms correctly: keep your elbows bent at a 90-degree angle and close to your sides, and swing your arms from the shoulders. As you step forward with your right foot, your left arm will pump forward and your right elbow will come straight behind your body so that your right hand almost brushes your right hip. When pumping your arms, don't let them come higher than chest level, and keep your hands relaxed in loose fists.

## Walk in Water

Head to the pool for a great cardiovascular workout that doesn't have to involve swimming. Walking in water is ideal if you have joint pain or arthritis, you're overweight, you've never exercised before, or you just want to do something different with your walking routine. Because the water provides resistance, this increases the amount of work your body has to do. Indeed, in a study at the Royal United Hospital in England, researchers found that walking in chest-deep water increased the participants' heart rate and oxygen consumption—both are measures of aerobic intensity—more than walking at the same pace on land.

How to do it: Stand in waist- or chest-deep water at one end of the pool with your arms out of the water. For the first step, lift your right foot high (almost as if you were marching) and place it on the pool bottom, landing with your heel, rolling through the foot, and pushing off with your toes; as you do this, your left arm will swing forward naturally, just as it would on land. For the next step, repeat this motion with the left foot and right arm. As you stride across the pool, keep your shoulders and trunk fairly still (don't twist) and stand tall (don't lean forward). Once you've mastered the technique, you can increase the difficulty by dropping your hands into the water and cupping them; as you swing the opposite arm and leg, your hands will create a whirlpool motion in the water, which increases the resistance your body must move through.

## QUIZ: *Do You Have the Right Fitness Goals?*

When it comes to embarking on an exercise program, it's better to be realistic than idealistic. Otherwise, you could be setting yourself up for a fall (perhaps literally) or serious disappointment. To find out which camp you belong to, answer the following questions True or False.

1. If you want to maximize your body's calorie-burning potential, you should do aerobic exercise exclusively.
2. The only way to get calm energy through exercise is to do yoga.
3. Interval training is a good way to crank up the intensity of your workouts without overexerting yourself.
4. If you want to know how hard you're exercising, you need to wear a heart-rate monitor.
5. To prevent injuries, you shouldn't increase the intensity or duration of your workouts by more than 25 percent each week.
6. For the sake of continuity, you shouldn't take off more than two days of exercise in a row.
7. Your workout time is better spent exercising at full throttle rather than wasting time on warming up or cooling down.
8. Strength training can help you slim down, just as aerobic exercise can.
9. You should always keep your strength-training sessions separate from your aerobic workouts.

10. It's better to frame your exercise goals in terms of the specific steps you'll actually take than in terms of the results you desire.

Scoring:

|     |       |       |
|-----|-------|-------|
| 1.  | T = 1 | F = 2 |
| 2.  | T = 1 | F = 2 |
| 3.  | T = 2 | F = 1 |
| 4.  | T = 1 | F = 2 |
| 5.  | T = 2 | F = 1 |
| 6.  | T = 2 | F = 1 |
| 7.  | T = 1 | F = 2 |
| 8.  | T = 2 | F = 1 |
| 9.  | T = 1 | F = 2 |
| 10. | T = 2 | F = 1 |

Now add up your score and see how you fared.

**17–20 points: You have the right stuff.** It looks as if you are well informed about what different forms of exercise can and can't do for you. Plus, you have realistic expectations about how to safely start an exercise program as well as a sense of what's reasonable to anticipate in the way of results. These are the essential ingredients for leading a more active lifestyle over the long run. Now you're ready to put them to good use.

**14–16 points: You have some of the right ideas.** Your fitness knowledge base is a bit inconsistent. Maybe that's because you're subscribing to some outdated ideas about the benefits of certain forms of exercise. Or maybe you're a little too gung ho for your own good. Give yourself a brief refresher course on the facts of a fit life and you'll be in a better spot for taking the exercise plunge.

**10–13 points: Your mind-set needs relocating.** It appears that you're in need of some reeducation about what's realistic to expect from various forms of exercise, as well as how to begin an exercise program safely. Brush up on the basics from this chapter and the previous one, and you'll be better able to protect yourself from painful injuries and dashed hopes.

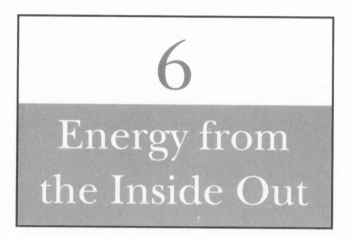

# 6

# Energy from the Inside Out

While being physically active can do wonders to boost your stamina, there's no denying that feeling blue can sap you of energy. There are numerous factors that can make you lethargic. My sister Jane observed about my once-destructive eating behaviors that after our parents divorced, I used to swallow up my hurt by overeating. Looking back, it's clear how reaching for food was my way to circumvent, rather than deal with, the real issues I was experiencing.

It's unfortunate that there's still such a stigma surrounding mental illness, and it's particularly tragic that people are still suffering from conditions that can easily be treated with medicine, such as depression. If you are always tired, you should see your doctor immediately. If you and your doctor have ruled out a medical basis for your fatigue, it may be time to assess your lifestyle and frame of mind. Beyond giving me a healthy diet, Weight Watchers truly helped restore my energy by giving me tools to cope with the emotional issues that had for years triggered my subtle acts of self-destruction.

When I'm feeling underenergized and overwhelmed, I try to go through a kind of mental deconstruction process whereby I take apart and examine the various facets of my life. There will always be things I can't control, and accepting that fact helps me to focus on the areas I really can control. As a single mother I need to work, but the kinds of work I take on are my choice. My career takes me away from my girls far more than I'd like, and there are times when I dread the thought of going off on another business trip. The upside is that I am proud of the work I do and lucky that I can schedule my commitments around school breaks, weekends, and holidays, thus giving us stretches of quality time together throughout the year. It still bothers me when the press runs stories about me that are exaggerated or untrue. My only recourse is to focus on what I know to be true, what I call "living in truth." Once at a dark moment in my life I asked a priest whether the truth about me would ever he heard over the constant lies reported by the media. He said that the truth would always prevail if I lived my life with truth in my heart. He was right, and the wisdom he shared with me that day changed me forever.

Negative thinking is, unquestionably, one of the most destructive forces in our lives. While it's impossible to hide our heads in the sand to avoid problems, there's plenty we can do to manage the amount of negativity in our day-to-day lives. Instead of exhausting myself trying to be everything to everyone, I now focus my life around key goals. I also surround myself with people whom I admire and who are supportive of me. Today I find myself drawn to positive-minded people, and this has made me think more optimistically. When I began working for Weight Watchers, my critics said it was undignified for me to promote dieting. In my eyes, I see my Weight Watchers work as an opportunity to speak out on a major health issue, and in recent years I've accomplished a great deal to raise awareness of the risks associated with obesity. I was proud when the American Heart Association approached me to be a national spokesperson, and I'm equally proud of the work I've been doing to have obesity prevention understood by legislators responsible for the nation's health policies. I'm truly energized by the health topics I discuss, knowing that the public

## KEEPING IN TOUCH

"I feel anxious when I leave the girls for more than a few days. I have to be careful to keep these feelings in check because even subtle anxiety will drain energy just as much as physical fatigue. Setting boundaries helps. I call home a few times each day, and I always take a few minutes to speak to the girls after school and again at bedtime. I like to fax them poems or sketches from my various hotel stops, too."

stage allows me to make a difference in people's lives. I've come a long way in recent years, but feelings of regret over the past still seem to rain on my parade.

I had the privilege to visit His Holiness the Dalai Lama last year when I was filming a documentary on spirituality for the BBC. I was almost speechless in the presence of this great and wise man, but I managed to ask him how I might come to terms with my past. Facing the palms of his hands one atop the other, he made a sweeping gesture, as if wiping a slate clean. He said there is no word in the Tibetan language for "guilt," which he likened to negative energy, and he explained that negativity is what prevents people from attaining harmony in their own lives. When I feel myself falling back into my formerly negative ways, I try to draw on this wisdom, which has helped lift a tremendous burden from my shoulders.

It's great to feel in control, but it's good to know you can learn a lot when things don't go according to plan. It's said that when life hands you lemons, you should make lemonade. In a way that's what I did on the morning I left Calcutta for the fifteen-hour train trip to Dharamsala, India, where the Dalai Lama resides. I'd arrived at the station quite late, and in the rush several of my bags were left back at the car, including my case filled with all the books and research notes I'd spent months gathering. I'd planned to read most of the way, and the mix-up left me feeling panicked and unprepared. There was nothing I could do, of course, and after much hand-wringing I resolved that at least I would sit back and enjoy the ride. Before long I was immersed in the incredible sights, sounds, and smells of the land and culture I'd come so far to visit. Only hours before, I had felt wasted by frustration, but now I was upbeat and invigorated as I chatted away with fellow passengers, making the most of my unexpected good fortune. Needless to say, I arrived feeling more excited than nervous and I was far better informed than if I'd buried my nose in my books.

# Energy and Your Emotions

If only your personal energy deficit could be completely cured by improving your eating habits, losing weight, or getting fit, life would be rather grand, wouldn't it? But there's more to the energy picture than these elements alone. Other aspects of your lifestyle and your personal habits can also affect the vitality you feel—for better or worse. Your diet could be absolutely pristine and your physical life vigorous, but if you don't support these practices with plenty of sleep or ample time to de-stress and rejuvenate your spiritual side, you won't be doing all that you can to bolster your energy.

After all, it's essential to take steps to increase your energy from the inside out, because the biggest energy drain in your life often lies in your head—in your habits. In other words, your emotional habits or your state of mind could be sabotaging your energy and causing you to feel sluggish. The secret of boosting your energy from the inside out is to mindfully engage in lifestyle practices that will bolster, rather than squander, your energy and to cultivate a positive mental attitude instead of letting negative thoughts deplete your sense of well-being. It's a matter of coming to your own emotional rescue, of throwing yourself a life raft that can bring you to a better place. Otherwise, you'll simply be working against yourself instead of being your own ally in the energy game.

Yet many women pour all their energy into what needs to get done—at work and at home, or for loved ones or their community—and as a result, they often have little energy left for themselves. Does this sound familiar? If so, this accidental martyrdom could be a problem for your sense of well-being and your goals. Consider the following: You want to clean up your lifestyle or lose weight, but you don't have the energy reserves to do it. Or you want to carve out more time for spiritual renewal so you'll feel more grounded in your everyday life, but your schedule is constantly overbooked. Where do these scenarios leave you? Right where you are now: feeling helpless, overwhelmed, and stuck in a rut. The truth is, feeling scattered or overcommitted can waste your energy by spreading it too thin. Feeling centered in your life, on the other hand, can help you direct your energy to where you really want it to go. When you feel as though you are in control of your life, your decisions and actions are likely to be much more efficient, which can help you use—and conserve—your energy wisely.

# Taking Care of Your Needs

Before you can feel centered, though, you'll need to know what you want and need in your life. The truth is, many women are so busy running around doing things for other people that they're out of touch with their own needs. This fact is precisely why it's important to regularly take stock of what you really want and need. The only way to do this is to dare to ask the crystallizing questions: What am I missing? What do I crave most in my life? What do I need in my life to feel more grounded? Once you have zeroed in on these factors, you can figure out which needs your partner can meet, which your friends can meet, which your job or community can meet, and which needs you can meet yourself.

As far as those needs you can provide for yourself, you'll need to practice healthy self-care, the potential benefits of which are enormous. Taking good psychological and emotional care of yourself can help shore up your self-esteem when it's flagging. It can make life seem more manageable and more enjoyable because it gives you breathing room. It can help improve the quality of your relationships by making you less needy or stressed out. And it can help replenish energy that's been spent on everyday activities—precious energy you'll need to maintain motivation to make the changes in your life that you want.

You might be wondering how in the world you're going to find the time to devote to self-care when you're perpetually short on free time. It's a valid question, and there's a simple answer: You need to start creating time to recharge your batteries and rejuvenate your spirit. It won't be easy to carve out private time at first, but it is essential for your sense of well-being. It can be done if you start setting limits with people and requests that have the potential to drain your energy; if you identify your true priorities and set up your schedule so that it reflects what's most important to you; if you strike a balance between pursuing your goals with energy and enthusiasm and taking time to replenish your reserves with a little R and R; and if you set aside personal time—that can be spent writing in a journal, painting or engaging in another cherished hobby, listening to music, or doing other activities that help you unwind and restore your own precious energy on a near-daily basis. Once you get in the habit of carving out this revitalizing time for yourself, you'll come to value it enormously, and you'll probably even guard it as if your energy depended on it—which it does.

# How to Stop the Busyness Epidemic

Many women have a tendency to be in perpetual motion, to commit to more projects than they can realistically—or sanely—handle. As a result, they wind up rushing to fulfill their myriad responsibilities, without feeling as though they're doing anything well enough. Not only can this deprive you of the satisfaction of a job well done, but it can make you feel vaguely disconnected from your life: when you're so busy simply trying to get everything done in a twenty-four-hour day, hurrying from one task to the next, the individual moments of your life often don't fully register. Over time, this pattern can wear you out.

Indeed, practice makes perfect when it comes to being hectic, exhausted, and energy-depleted. How can you stop the cycle? By taking an unvarnished look at your life and evaluating whether how you're spending your time jibes with what's truly important to you—in other words, by getting off the carousel at least long enough to think about what you're doing with your actions. This way you can reassess whether you're living your life according to your priorities—or whether you're simply setting yourself up to crash and burn at regular intervals.

Before you say yes to the next project, invitation, or request, ask yourself these four questions:

1. Do I really want to do this—and, if so, why?
2. Do I really have the time to do this?
3. Will my life be significantly enriched if I do this?
4. What might be the personal payoff if I said no?

Once you've asked yourself these questions, weigh your answers against each other and let the balance determine your decision. Doing this exercise on a regular basis will help you avoid overextending yourself and spending energy needlessly. Instead, you can use the extra time to regroup and recharge your batteries.

# Putting the Brakes on Sacrificing Sleep

Without a doubt, skimping on sleep ranks at the top of the list of culprits that could be robbing you of energy. After all, we're in the midst of an epidemic of sleep deprivation: These days, the average adult sleeps six hours and fifty-four minutes a night during the week, according to the National Sleep Foundation, even though sleep experts generally recommend eight hours of shut-eye per night. Granted, it's tempting to try to capture more time to catch up on uncompleted tasks late at night, but skimping on sleep will come back to haunt you. Those lost hours of precious slumber can add up until you begin to feel as though you're dragging yourself through the day.

Over time, this discrepancy between the sleep you need and the sleep you actually get can have serious consequences for your health and your life. Not only can losing sleep increase your risk of work-related accidents or having a car accident—moderate sleep loss has been shown to impair coordination as much as being legally drunk—but it may also compromise your immune function, your speech, your mood, your memory, and your cognitive performance. What's more, a study from the University of Chicago suggests that carrying a chronic sleep debt may adversely affect carbohydrate metabolism and endocrine function, setting you up for possible weight gain. Plus, cheating yourself of precious sleep can make you feel more irritable, aggressive, and out of sorts on a daily basis.

The bottom line: it's just not worth it to burn the candle at both ends and sacrifice sleep in order to take on more work, family, or social obligations. What you should do, instead, is to honor your true sleep needs. You can figure out how much sleep you personally require by conducting an experiment. Choose a stretch of three to five days—such as during vacation—when you don't have to wake up at a particular time. Go to bed at your usual time, then sleep until you wake up naturally—meaning without an alarm. Because most people carry a sleep debt, it may take you a few days to catch up on lost sleep and figure out how much slumber you actually need each night. After three to five days, you can use the last night's sleep as an indication of your true needs. Aim to get that much on a regular basis by moving your bedtime fifteen minutes earlier each week until you can establish a pattern of going to bed at the same time each night and awakening at the same time each morning, while still getting all the zzzs you need.

Of course, it's also crucial to set yourself up for good quality sleep. Most people have a rough night every now and then, and it's usually nothing to worry about. But sleeping poorly night after night can compromise your ability to function physically, mentally, and emotionally. To gain better snooze control, you'll need to practice good sleep hygiene. Here's how:

## Stick with a Consistent Sleep Schedule
The body's internal clock craves consistency and predictability, so your ability to fall asleep and stay asleep depends on your schedule. If you tend to go to bed or wake up at irregular times, your brain may not be in sync with your erratic schedule, which means you might end up lying in bed, counting sheep when you want to be slumbering. What's more, a study at Brigham and Women's Hospital in Boston found that even people who

get enough sleep are likely to be irritable or downbeat if they wake up at a time other than what they're used to.

### Avoid Unnecessary Stimulation
Steer clear of caffeine and cigarettes late in the day as well as alcohol, which can make you drowsy initially but could cause you to wake up in the wee hours of the night.

### Move Your Body During the Day
Most sleep experts agree that exercising moderately on a regular basis—whether by walking briskly, jogging, cycling, swimming, or doing aerobics—can help enhance the quality of sleep by causing a rise in body temperature, followed by a fall around bedtime (which has a soporific effect). Just don't exercise too close to bedtime; try to allow at least three hours after your workout before turning in.

### Eat Lightly in the Evening
Consuming a heavy meal before bedtime can increase alertness or give you middle-of-the-night indigestion. Have a light dinner, and if you tend to wake up hungry during the night, have a sleep-friendly snack such as a small bowl of cereal with milk or a cup of chamomile tea and some graham crackers.

### Create a Dreamy Bedroom Environment
It's no surprise that noise can disturb sleep, so if you live near a busy intersection or airport, you may want to buy some earplugs or drown out unwanted sounds with a white-noise machine or a tape of a soothing sound, such as a running stream. Similarly, if excess light seeps through your windows from the street, consider splurging on heavier curtains or blackout shades. A firm mattress and pillow can also help, but make sure your pillow isn't so high that it throws your neck out of alignment.

### Relax Before Bedtime
Don't watch the 11 o'clock news. Take a warm bath, meditate, do deep-breathing and stretching exercises, or read an enjoyable (but not too stimulating) book. The goal is to quiet your mind and set yourself up for a night of restful sleep.

It may seem like a monumental task to revamp your evening habits, but it's worth the effort. If you improve the quality of your sleep, you're likely to wake up the next morning feeling better refreshed and more buoyant. And if you feel as though you have more physical and emotional energy, you'll be in a better position to improve your eating and exercise habits—or to tackle other challenges in your life.

# Fatigue Factors You Can Fix

Once you've addressed and improved your sleeping patterns, you'll probably begin to feel more restored in body, mind, and spirit, which can make you feel more energized in your waking hours. But don't forget about your daytime habits. After all, how you conduct yourself during the daylight hours can also affect your sense of vim and vigor. Here are four potential energy robbers you'll want to catch and fix.

## Walking Around in a Slump

Poor posture doesn't just make you look tired; it creates the feeling as well, because when the spine and joints aren't properly aligned the body has to work that much harder just to get around. Think of energy as flowing through your body similar to the way water flows through a hose: if there are any unnecessary bends or crimps in the pipeline, the energy won't flow as smoothly or plentifully as it should.

The solution: Stand tall—and proud. While standing, keep your head lined up over—not in front of—your body, your ears directly over your shoulders, your shoulders directly over your hips, and your knees over your toes. Your knees shouldn't be locked, and your feet should be hip width apart. Aim to create one line from the top of your head to the base of your feet, as if you had a pole pulling you upright from the center of your body. Keeping your spine and your joints in their proper alignment can make you feel strong and competent; plus, it's less likely to strain your muscles or tire your body out.

## Waiting to Inhale or Exhale Fully

Many women make a habit of breathing shallowly without even realizing it. The problem is, when you breathe shallowly, you don't end up taking in enough oxygen; as a result, you're likely to have lower levels of oxygen and higher levels of carbon dioxide in your blood than you should—which can make you feel tired. What to do: practice breathing from your diaphragm. To see if you're doing this correctly, place your hand over your belly button. As you inhale, your abdomen and chest should rise about an inch; as you exhale, they should fall about an inch. You should be able to feel this rising and falling motion with your hand. Take breaks from what you're doing and practice this several times per day—and soon breathing deeply will come naturally.

## Living Like a Mushroom

Depriving yourself of natural sunlight may protect your skin from the sun's harmful rays, but it won't do your state of mind much good. Without periodic exposure to natural light, your brain and body will go into sleep mode. Some people are especially sensitive to light deprivation; if they don't get enough light, they get depressed or tired. This is why seasonal affective disorder (SAD) typically occurs in the winter months, which tend to have less natural light and fewer hours of daylight. The antidote: bright lights. Research has found that regular bright-light exposure can improve the symptoms, including fatigue and sadness, of both SAD and PMS. The upshot: seek the light whenever possible. Sneak outside for a ten-minute walk at least once during the day; even on a cloudy day, you'll get considerably more light exposure than you would in an office, for example. If getting outside is absolutely impossible, at least go into a room that's filled with natural light for a few minutes. As a third resort, it may help to spend about ten minutes in a brightly lit room such as the bathroom (if you have vanity lights).

## Keeping Your Nose to the Grindstone All Day

This may earn points with your boss, but it won't with your energy level. Staying in one position for long periods of time can sap your energy because your circulation slows down; plus, your body naturally associates stillness with sleep, which puts you in the mood to snooze. The remedy is simple: get up and walk around for at least a few minutes every now and then. Your body will appreciate the movement, and your mind will appreciate the break from whatever it is you were doing. Chances are, you'll return to the task feeling energized.

# Dealing with Stress

There's no question that the amount of energy you feel can be a reflection of your state of mind, as well as your habits. If you feel happy and excited about what's happening in your life, you'll probably feel physically and emotionally buoyant, and you'll have energy to spare. But if you're bogged down with worry, anxiety, guilt, or other negative emotions, you probably won't have much pep in your step or in your outlook.

Stress certainly gets a bad name in the energy equation—and deservedly so. But not all stress is created equal. In fact, there is a form of stress that can actually be beneficial: it's called prostress, and it is defined as "the positive, psychological state you experience when you perceive a situation as challenging, potentially pleasurable in some way, and as offering positive consequences such as growth, desired change, or accomplishment of a goal," according to psychologist Simone Ravica, Ph.D., author of *High on Stress: A Woman's Guide to Optimizing the Stress in Her Life* (New Harbinger). With negative stress (aka distress), you tend to feel helpless or frustrated because a situation is out of your control (or at least feels that way). With positive stress (or prostress), you perceive a situation as a challenge rather than a threat, so you feel motivated and stimulated to do whatever you can to improve the situation's outcome—or at least to learn or grow from the experience of trying.

Ideally, you want to minimize the amount of negative stress and maximize the amount of positive stress in your life. Of course, you can't always choose one form over the other, but you can tilt the balance somewhat by tinkering with your perceptions. After all, how you perceive and react to stress—both good and bad—is largely within your control. So if you can train yourself to stop overreacting to negative stress (such as traffic jams or computer glitches) and save that energy and pour it into the pursuit of positive challenges (such as exercising or losing weight), your state of mind will be much improved and so will your sense of vitality. If you do this on a continuous basis, you'll gradually gain a can-do spirit and a feeling of empowerment that will, in turn, fuel a greater sense of optimism and energy.

Admittedly, it's not as easy as making a conscious switch from negative to positive stress. But you can change the way you typically deal with stress—namely, by becoming more proactive and less reactive. Your first step is to think about the situation at hand—whether it involves a testy boss, a household disaster, or an alarmingly high credit card bill—and ask yourself these questions:

- Can you change the situation?
- Should you try to change it?
- If so, how threatening or urgent is the situation?
- If you can actually do something about it—and it's worth the effort—map out a plan of action.

On the other hand, if you can't do anything about the situation, you may need to look at what you can do to improve how you're feeling. This is where strategies that are designed to change your physical and emotional reaction to a particular source of stress come in: engaging in meditation, yoga, or deep-breathing exercises, smelling soothing scents, or listening to calming music on a regular basis can help calm your physical and emotional responses to a stressful event.

Or you can use visualization techniques to quell your reaction to stress: imagine the irritating factor being encapsulated in a balloon and floating up into the sky until it disappears—or imagine simply shutting the irritating factor in the closet. Sometimes it pays not to struggle endlessly with a problem until you can come up with a solution. After all, research has found that ruminating or dwelling on problems increases your risk of depression; in fact, the tendency to ruminate is decidedly female, which may be one reason why women are twice as likely to suffer depression as men are. Sometimes you're better off simply letting a problem go if it doesn't have a ready-made answer. That way you can channel the energy you would have spent on that stressful issue into something you can actually do something about. And you never know, sometimes the vexing problems find a way to resolve themselves; or a solution may unexpectedly arrive at a later date. In the meantime, you will have spared yourself the stress of mulling it over again and again.

## Talk Therapy for Your Energy

While you're revamping the way you respond to stress, you should also take an honest look at the way you talk to yourself. The truth is, we all talk to ourselves on a regular basis, and this running commentary typically revolves around the challenges we face or our ability to handle them. Yet often people don't even realize that their inner voice is speaking; they simply accept the message as fact. Psychologists call this inner dialogue self-talk, and they have found that what you tell yourself can have a profound effect, for better or worse, on how you feel, what you do, and how you see the world. And because it can color your entire outlook, self-talk can affect your energy level as well as what you do with it.

Depending on the content of these internal messages, they can either help or hinder your performance and your ability to reach your goals. Positive self-talk—having an internal voice that's upbeat, encouraging, and constructive—can help you feel more confident and focused in everyday life; it can provide you with sustainable motivation and encouragement to tackle new challenges and persist in the face of setbacks. On the other hand, negative self-talk—namely, being overly critical of yourself, predicting doom or disaster, blaming or simply saying nasty things to yourself—can be downright detrimental to your well-being and your energy level. It's like having an abusive parrot on your shoulder, constantly putting you down.

The best way to get rid of self-critical habits is to pay attention to what you say to yourself on a regular basis and change it when necessary. Once you become attuned to the negative or discouraging things you say to yourself, correct those misguided thoughts and replace them with more positive, constructive, or at least neutral messages. It might help to jot down the negative things you say to yourself for three consecutive days and make a note of what was going on when your inner critic chimed in. After you become aware of patterns to what you say to yourself and when, make a concerted effort to let a more encouraging internal voice stick up for you or spur you along. Use statements such as "I can" or "I will" when describing your intentions. Counter self-flagellation with a re-ality check when you make a mistake. Use positive affirmations to remind yourself that you are capable of achieving your goal and that you deserve to succeed. If you want the more constructive, upbeat style to come naturally, you'll need to practice this positive self-talk—and eliminate the negative form—on a regular basis. It's a matter of retraining your mind, which can, in turn, reinvigorate your body's pep.

## FAST FIXES FOR ENERGY-DRAINING EMOTIONS

Could it be that your emotions are squandering your energy? If you have any of the following habits, you've just been put on notice that you may be sabo-taging your vitality. What you'll want to do, in that case, is banish the emotions that are zapping your zest and replace them with more helpful habits:

**BEING CONSUMED WITH ANGER:** It's not just bad for your health. Anger can kill your energy, too, because with chronic anger, stress hormones—such as adrena-line and cortisol—are flowing all the time, which takes a toll on your body. You just can't stay in that fight-or-flight position for very long without feeling burnt out. **The energizing answer:** Learn to manage your anger by making a conscious decision about what's worth getting mad about. Ask yourself, "Is this petty stuff?" If so, take some deep breaths or do another relaxation exercise and picture your anger evaporating like a bottle of uncapped perfume.

**WORRYING ABOUT WHAT COULD HAPPEN:** When you repeatedly think about lots of things that could go wrong, you wind up expending lots of mental and emo-tional energy without actually doing anything productive. Plus, worrying can make you so preoccupied that you don't enjoy the good things that happen that could recharge you. **A better tactic:** Set worry hours—say, half an hour in the late after-noon—and worry your heart out about everything you can think of. Try to think of constructive solutions, then put these issues out of your mind.

**FEELING GUILTY:** When you start second-guessing yourself or constantly ques-tion who you are and what you're doing, it's exhausting; in essence, it's like yelling at yourself all the time. **How to bag the guilt?** Listen to what you're saying to your-self and think about where it came from. Then ask yourself if it's true. If it isn't, the guilt is likely to vanish naturally. If it is, you can then do something about it, if you choose to.

**HOLDING YOURSELF TO PERFECTIONISTIC STANDARDS:** If this is your m.o., nothing you do will ever be good enough so you'll continue to strive and strive—to no avail. After all, perfectionism is unattainable. **The solution:** Strive for excellence instead of perfection. Do the best you can on whatever it is you have to do, then let it go.

**REVISITING BAD TIMES—AGAIN AND AGAIN:** Research from San Jose State University in California has found that dwelling on negative events from the past is associated with lower stamina, whereas looking forward to the future is associated with higher stamina. **Your perspective prescription:** Put the past in its place and focus on what you can do to make your life meaningful and enjoyable today and tomorrow.

# Relaxing to Rejuvenate

It may sound counterintuitive, but one of the best ways to revitalize your energy is to practice relaxation exercises on a regular basis. Not only do these techniques give you a minivacation from the chaos of the modern world, but they can help unclutter your mind, soothe your body, and promote a physical and mental sense of calm that can help replenish your spent energy reserves. Quite simply, relaxation techniques such as meditation are the equivalent of an antidote to stress. Indeed, more and more research is suggesting that meditation, in particular, is good medicine for your mind, body, and soul. It can lower high blood pressure, improve symptoms of irritable bowel syndrome, reduce pain, and ease anxiety, among other conditions. What's more, research by the Center for Health and Aging Studies at Maharishi University in Fairfield, Iowa, has found that transcendental meditation can counter the effects of stress on the body—namely, by decreasing the amount of cortisol that's released during a stressful experience.

The reason meditation is so effective is that it produces what Herbert Benson, M.D., of Harvard Medical School calls a "relaxation response"— a physiological state of profound calm, the opposite of the fight-or-flight response that's sparked by stress. There are many ways to achieve this response—you can practice yoga, qi gong, walking, or prayer, for example—but meditation has been one of the more widely studied routes. While there are different forms of meditation—such as transcendental meditation and mindfulness meditation—many involve a combination of sitting quietly, focusing on your breathing, and repeating a word or phrase. Here's how to do one variation, favored by Dr. Benson; just follow these six steps:

1. Find a quiet room, sit in a comfortable position, and close your eyes.
2. Relax your muscles, starting with your feet and slowly progressing up to your calves, thighs, abdomen, chest, shoulders, head, and neck.
3. Breathe slowly and naturally, and repeat a soothing word (such as "serendipity"), a sound (whoosh), or a prayer (you're on your own with this one) silently to yourself as you exhale.
4. When distracting thoughts come to mind, simply disregard them and focus on the repetition. Continue this for ten to twenty minutes.
5. Afterwards, sit quietly for another minute or so and allow thoughts to reenter your mind. Recognize how much calmer and more in control you feel, then stand up and move on.
6. If you do this once or twice a day, you'll silence the chaos within your mind and body. And in all likelihood, you'll gain a feeling of calm, focused energy.

Just as it's essential to fuel your body's energy with good eating and exercise habits, it's vital that you nourish and nurture your emotional needs for the sake of your psyche and your spirit. The goal is to get off the stress roller coaster and reclaim control over how you move, breathe, think, and run your life so that you can energize yourself. It's a matter of putting an end to running on adrenaline and allowing yourself to cultivate calm, focused energy instead. This will help your body recharge its batteries and help you handle your life more efficiently, which will likely give you time and energy to spare. Then you can pour that newfound energy into honoring your personal needs and revitalizing your spiritual side. This is energy well spent because it will help you attain your goals, fulfill your dreams, and enhance your well-being.

## NINE WAYS TO GET INSTANT ENERGY

Sometimes the need to pep yourself up can seem especially urgent. In that case, it's all well and good to strive for long-term energy, but what you also need is a quick boost at the moment. Fortunately, you may be able to fight your fatigue and bolster your energy with some fast-acting tricks. Even if some of these aren't rooted in hard science, they may be worth a try if you're craving an energy boost. After all, what have you got to lose—except, perhaps, your sluggishness?

1. **Take a whiff of peppermint or jasmine.** It's not just your imagination: these bracing scents may increase the beta waves in your brain, stimulating alertness.

2. **Visualize your energy.** Remember a time when you felt highly energized—during an exhilarating hike, for example—and try to recapture that feeling in the way you move.

3. **Wear something red.** Because red is the color of fire, it spurs you to action by causing a rise in blood pressure and heart rate, the release of adrenaline, and stimulation of the brain, according to Leatrice Eiseman, director of the Pantone Color Institute and author of *Colors for Your Every Mood* (Capital Books).

4. **Indulge in a yawn.** Because it delivers a blast of oxygen to the blood and the brain, it can actually boost mental alertness.

5. **Have a good laugh.** Not only does laughter reduce stress, anxiety, and worry, but it also increases heart rate, circulation, and oxygen consumption, all of which can give you a surge of energy. More good reasons to read the comics!

6. **Listen to invigorating music.** Faster, high-pitched music in major keys (such as Vivaldi's *The Four Seasons*) tends to foster brighter moods, according to Pierce J. Howard, Ph.D., director of research for the Center for Applied Cognitive Studies in Charlotte, North Carolina.

7. **Put on a high-wattage smile.** Research has found that when people smile and place a pleasant expression on their faces, this can actually affect their mood for the better. In other words, the act can spark the genuine feeling—and before you know it, you'll actually be in an upbeat mood.

8. **Take a short nap.** A brief nap, from twenty to thirty minutes, in the midafternoon can do wonders for your alertness and energy level, especially if you nap regularly and for the same amount of time. But napping is likely to backfire if you suffer from insomnia, so don't sleep during the day if you have trouble sleeping well at night.

9. **Have a chat with a vibrant friend.** Yes, energy can be contagious. Spend a little time with an enthusiastic, high-energy person, and chances are some of her natural buoyancy will rub off on you. Plus, socializing can help you shift gears and take your mind off your worries for a while.

If you're truly serious about wanting to pump up your energy, you may need to look beneath the surface of your life at what could be robbing your zest. To find out whether your habits, habitat, or head are squandering your resources, answer the following questions Yes or No.

1. Are you bored or "underchallenged" in your job?
2. Is your home or office disorganized?
3. Do you routinely cut back on sleep to eke more hours out of each day?
4. Do you live in a noisy environment?
5. Do you often spend all day indoors?
6. Do you frequently worry about "what ifs" and other problems that could happen?
7. Do you have a tendency to take on more than you can comfortably handle?
8. Are you often so busy catering to other people's needs that you're out of touch with your own?
9. Do you often self-medicate—with food or alcohol, for example—to cope with stress?
10. Do you often feel as though other people's moods drag you down?

Now, give yourself one point for each time you answered Yes. If you scored:

**6–10 points:** You're setting yourself up to crash and burn. Of course you're tired—how could you not be? Between everything that you're doing and the lack of positive support or stimulation you're experiencing in your life, your routine is blasting your energy into smithereens before you have a chance to use it the way you want to. It's time for you to come to your own rescue—by revamping your environment and/or how you deal with stress. Review this chapter and seek new ways to take charge of your life—in energy-enhancing ways.

**3–5 points:** You're letting precious energy slip away in subtle ways. Your lifestyle is supporting your energy-promoting goals to a certain extent. But some of your energy is slipping away unnoticed. Maybe it's because you're caught up in the busyness epidemic and you're always on the go, even when you don't need to be. Or maybe you're cheating yourself of restorative sleep too often. Look for new opportunities to lighten your load of responsibilities and commitments and strive to achieve a balance between satisfying your needs and other people's.

0–2 points: **Your lifestyle is supporting your energy.** Whether through sheer luck or smart work on your part, the circumstances of your life are energy-friendly, and so are many of your habits. Your best bet is to keep up the status quo—without resting on your laurels. Indeed, you'd be wise to take stock of your needs and wants periodically and to come up with novel strategies to cultivate more premium-quality energy in your life. You won't regret the effort.

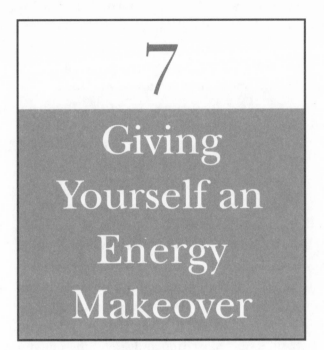

# 7

# Giving Yourself an Energy Makeover

In the previous chapters we've focused a great deal on the physical aspects of energizing our lives. We've said that one of the biggest benefits of a healthy lifestyle built on good nutrition, adequate exercise, and a positive mind-set is the energy to keep up with all the things we need to do. As much as I like feeling productive and purposeful, I no longer feel that all of my energy should be spent on work alone. My life would not be nearly as full or exciting had I not learned to devote some of my energy to doing the things I do purely for pleasure.

For example, I love writing, watercolor painting, and photography; and Pilates also invigorates me. Even simple pleasures such as lighting a log fire or just sipping a cup of hot tea have the power to replenish and renew what an active life drains away. Today I manage to participate in them all to some degree. These outlets do more than just relax me; they challenge and fulfill me in unique and important ways.

Yoga has taught me to channel my energy, and now I find it vital to maintaining my energy bank. I used to take breathing for granted, for example, but through yoga I now understand its effect on my mind, body, and soul.

Expressing my ideas through words and images excites me, and producing something beautiful or provocative can be deeply gratifying. The *process* of creating can be exciting as well as relaxing, and I often wonder what I was thinking of back in the days when I'd abandoned pencils and paints for lack of energy. *Now they're among the tools that keep me energized!*

I've also discovered that something as natural and automatic as how I breathe can have a big effect on my mood and energy level. Our bodies respond almost instantly to each breath we take, which is why breathing too fast or too shallow when feeling stressed only makes matters worst. The antidote I've found can be to quite literally stop and take "a breather"—a few quiet moments during which I stop and restart my breathing with slow deep breaths. I do this by fully exhaling slowly and evenly through my nose. Just slowing my breathing has a relaxing and energizing effect on my body and mind, and in a few minutes I can move on with a clear and level head.

I think that taking risks from time to time also keeps me energized. Try something dramatically new and different, and who knows what will happen? I got my start as a children's book author after I decided to learn to fly to feel closer to my husband, whose career as a navy pilot kept him far from home. The technical aspects of pilot training could be a real grind for me, but the upside was that my imagination soared when I was out at the airfield. The surroundings inspired the artist and storyteller in me, and I started writing and sketching out stories about my training helicopter, whom I called "Budgie," and the menagerie of other planes in the hangar. The girls loved hearing my "Adventures of Budgie" before bedtime, but honestly, the idea of publishing them never occurred to me until a family friend encouraged me to give it a go.

It's said you are never too old to learn something new. To that I'd like to add that it's never too late to rediscover your passions. Whether it's needlepoint, swimming laps, or volunteer work that used to rev you up, do make a commitment to reintroduce yourself to a cherished pastime. Start doing things that take you away from the daily grind, and you'll find yourself feeling renewed again and again.

## RELAXING RITUALS

"Sometimes the littlest break can be a real pick-me-up. I carry a tube of a favorite scented cream in my handbag because I find its fragrance relaxing and invigorating. I light scented candles in the evening and even take some with me when I travel. The act of lighting the candle, combined with the soft light and delicate scent, helps me unwind after a tiring day."

# Making Changes in Your Life

There's no question that most of us live our lives almost exclusively in the fast lane these days. We've become highly successful at being hectic. We're pros at packing as many activities into our days and nights as is humanly possible. But what often happens when we continuously operate in this manner is that the incredibly savvy voice inside each of us—the one that cautions "Don't take on that extra project!" or "You need to slow down and get more rest!"—is drowned out in the drone of our busy, noisy lives. As a result, we become so task- and efficiency-oriented that we forget to take time to recharge our batteries. And we wind up getting into our own way when it comes to living a balanced life. Not surprisingly, that's when energy starts to feel like a shockingly ephemeral commodity.

Indeed, being a perpetual blur of motion and constantly going can eventually take a toll on your feelings of vitality, and it's important to slow down long enough to take stock of what you're doing and how you're spending your hours. Sometimes cultivating more energy requires doing less by paring back on your activities and returning to the basics of healthy living: eating well, exercising regularly, sleeping enough, having enough pleasure in your life, taking time to relax and rejuvenate yourself, and so on. It's a matter of redefining how you want to structure your life by placing your values and your energy concerns front and center rather than in the background.

You may need to shift your priorities and say no to some obligations or requests so that you can carve out time to restore your energy and revive your spirits. You may be forced to be more selective about whom you spend time with and reevaluate the value of your current occupation or other activities you regularly engage in, if they take too much out of you. Indeed, if some aspects of your life are continuous drains on your energy and you don't reap gratification from them, it may be worth removing or changing them.

Granted, it won't be easy to make these shifts at first, especially if change has been a foreign concept in your life so far, but getting more energy doesn't have to be as difficult as it may sound, either. It is possible to make lifestyle changes that will boost your energy without turning your life completely upside down. The key is to start slowly and gradually make changes in your diet or exercise habits or other lifestyle factors. After all, the goal is to make changes that you can live with and sustain—not changes that are going to make your life harder in the long run and hence become yet another drain on your energy.

As you continue your quest for more energy, your energy journal (see page 23) will

# Steering Clear of Energy Vampires

**B**e careful that you don't spend to much time with people who drain your energy. Some people call these types energy vampires; others call them toxic people or perpetual complainers. By any name, needy or self-centered friends, colleagues, and family members can drag down your spirits and suck the energy right out of you with their demands, complaints, or negativity.

The truth is, you can catch the moods of those around you, and this transmission can happen in a matter of seconds. That's because during conversation, we all naturally tend to synchronize our movements, posture, facial expressions, and speech rhythms to match the other person's, often without realizing it. In the process, we come to feel what the other person is feeling. There's been some suggestion that women may be especially vulnerable to this phenomenon, perhaps because we're better able to tune into and read other people's emotions and body language.

Since you can catch both negative and positive emotions, why not set yourself up to be happy as often as possible? Your best bet is to limit the time you spend with those who deplete your emotional energy, whenever possible, and choose to spend more time with friends and family members who are upbeat and supportive. They'll be more likely to rejuvenate you and lift your spirits. And the more you surround yourself with vigorous, positive people, the more vital and buoyant you're likely to feel.

become invaluable; it becomes your best friend because it will allow you to track the effects of your actions. This way, you can jot down notes about your revamped eating and exercise habits, how much sleep you're getting, how you're spending your time, and how these factors influence your energy level and state of mind. By monitoring these elements, you'll be able to see connections between what you're doing and how you're feeling. If you feel especially upbeat and energized for a couple of days, it's a good idea to review the preceding days to gauge what lifestyle or emotional factors may have contributed to that zestful feeling. Likewise, when you feel unusually lethargic, that's a good time to peruse your journal for clues about what made you feel that way.

Once you have a good pulse on these connections, you can set priorities for how you'll handle things differently in many areas of your life. It's rather like putting together the pieces of your own energy-boosting puzzle. You might vow to sneak in naps, for example, when you feel unusually tired or to give up your afternoon cookie and go for a revitalizing walk instead. You might decide to sign up for a yoga or meditation class after work instead of joining colleagues for a gripe session during happy hour. You might opt to spend more time in the evening playing games with your kids instead of vegetating in front of the television. What you want to do is identify what seems to be missing from your life—whether it's enough fun, adequate rest, or something else altogether—then to find ways to sneak more of that essential element in. Making these efforts will help you rebound from fatigue and return to a more energetic state.

## READING YOUR ENERGY METER

When you start changing your habits to change your energy level, you need to start paying attention to what's going on with your body and mind. Otherwise, how will you know what needs invigorating? Take short breaks during the day to check in with yourself and see how you're feeling. Use the following survey as a guide to gauging your energy level.

DO A QUICK BODY SCAN: Are you experiencing tension in your neck, your shoulders, or anywhere else in your body? Check your breathing—is it smooth and fairly deep or choppy and shallow? Are you slouching your way through the day or standing tall?

CHECK IN WITH YOUR THOUGHTS: Are you feeling frazzled, stressed out, or anxious? Does it seem as if you have a negative chatterbox in your mind? Or are you feeling calm and collected?

REVIEW YOUR RECENT REFUELING HISTORY: Have you had enough sleep recently? When was the last time you ate or drank something? Have you been sitting still for a substantial period of time?

Once you know the answers to these questions, you'll have a better sense of whether your energy level needs to be pumped up—and, if so, how to do it.

# Working with Your Natural Rhythms

To a certain extent, cycles of fatigue and energy are a normal part of life. And you may be able to plan some of the activities in your day so that they correspond to the natural peaks and valleys in muscle strength, alertness, and concentration that you're likely to experience at different hours. Indeed, when it comes to making the most of your energy, timing counts. Your body's circadian rhythms—the natural twenty-four-hour sleep-wake cycles and body chemistry fluctuations that are controlled by the body's internal clock—affect how alert, coordinated, sensitive, or physically strong you are throughout the day. To some degree, it's possible to use your natural highs to your advantage by arranging your schedule so that you can accomplish tasks you've set as priorities during your peak performance times.

Here's a look at how your hours of power stack up against each other and how you can put them to good use.

### Midmorning (9 to 11 A.M.)

Mental energy—in the form of mental acuity, short-term memory, logical reasoning skills, and concentration—peaks. As a result, this is a good time to tackle the day's most mentally challenging tasks: writing a report, balancing your checkbook, enduring a potentially stressful meetings.

### High Noon (12 P.M.)

Complex decision-making abilities hit their high point, which means this may be a good time to schedule a meeting in which important decisions must be made on the spot.

### Midafternoon (2 to 4 P.M.)

Your mental alertness and ability to concentrate may hit a slump between 2 and 3 P.M., whereas your coordination may actually improve between 2:30 and 4 P.M. As a result, this is a good window of opportunity for playing tennis or golf or typing a long report. But it's not the best time to try to concentrate on a complex task such as learning a new computer program.

### Late Afternoon (4 to 6 P.M.)

Muscle strength as well as aerobic and anaerobic capacities tend to peak in the late afternoon, according to research. That's why this may be a golden opportunity for scheduling a challenging workout, whether it involves strength-training or aerobic activities such as walking, running, biking, or swimming.

*Evening (6 to 8 P.M.)*

Sensory appreciation is most acute, but mental energy tends to trail off. As a result, this is a prime time for enjoying a favorite food, listening to pleasant music, or savoring a glass of fine wine—all of which can help you unwind after a taxing day. It's not an ideal time, however, to try to resolve complex family issues.

Once you become aware of these natural ebbs and flows in physical and mental vigor, you can seize opportunities to make the most of your abilities. It's a matter of strategic planning and smart scheduling. While this won't actually enhance your energy, it can help you make the most of the energy you have.

# Respecting Your Fatigue

Even with the best-laid plans for maximizing your energy, there will be times when you will feel quite tired. And it's important to remember that you need to heed your fatigue whenever it does make a forceful appearance that lasts more than a few hours; it's trying to tell you something. Maybe your energy balance is off kilter because you're not eating well, exercising wisely, sleeping or relaxing enough, or having enough fun in your life. Or maybe your body is fighting an illness and you need to keep a low profile or slip into low gear for a little while. Whatever is at the root of this fatigue, it is solvable—if you follow the advice you've been reading in this book. Perhaps you need to:

- **Upgrade your eating habits.** Practice portion control; consume plenty of fruits, vegetables, and whole-grain foods and some lean protein; and drink lots of water.
- **Shed excess pounds.** If you're overweight and low on energy, losing weight will surely boost your physical stamina and sense of vitality.
- **Clean up energy-draining habits.** If you smoke, quit; put an end to poor posture and shallow breathing; vow to get rid of your constant complaining or penchant for self-criticism.
- **Start moving regularly.** Embark on a regular exercise program that incorporates aerobic activities and strength training; also, try to sneak more movement into your everyday life.
- **Get smart about sleep.** Try to set up your schedule so that you can regularly get enough good-quality sleep for your personal needs.

- **Set aside sacred time to de-stress and rejuvenate.** Meditate; do yoga or qi gong; or practice deep-breathing or visualization exercises on a regular basis to restore your sense of equilibrium.
- **Nurture yourself with spiritual renewal.** Spend time in nature; paint, sculpt, or write poetry; play the piano or the guitar; discover the pursuits that bring you spiritual pleasure and renew your enthusiasm for life.

It's important to refuel your zest for life in all aspects of your life—physically, emotionally/psychologically, and spiritually—because each domain affects the others. When you feel depleted of emotional energy, for example, you're likely to feel physically tired as well. When you cheat yourself of private time to rejuvenate your spirit, it can take a toll on your physical and emotional well-being, too. After all, these various forms of energy have a synergistic effect. Just as your body, mind, and spirit are all housed in the same home that is you—and hence can affect one another's welfare, for better or worse—the same is true of your energy.

On the positive side, when you begin to take care of your physical, emotional, and spiritual energy, improvements in one domain can spur enhancements in the others. Consume a high-quality diet in moderate portions and get plenty of sleep on a regular basis, and you'll be providing yourself with ample fuel for an exercise program. Carve out time for essential relaxation, and you'll be on the road to minimizing the effects of stress on your body—and your physical energy reserves. And if you lose weight, which will relieve your physical fatigue, you'll likely feel a psychological boost as well. In fact, a study at Brown University School of Medicine in Providence, Rhode Island, found that after twenty-six obese people participated successfully in a twenty-six-week weight-loss program, they experienced a significant improvement in their sense of self-efficacy and self-confidence, giving them the courage to strive for what they wanted. The participants also experienced an elevation in their mood and physical comfort. So if you've been carrying around unwanted pounds, you might do well to start your energy makeover by slimming down, because this could create a cascade of energy-boosting changes in your life.

# A Three-Step Approach to
# Relieving Mental Fatigue

There's no question: it can be downright difficult to establish new habits when you're bogged down with apathy or stuck in a motivational rut. What you need to do, in that situation, is bust out of the rut and jump-start your motivation. This three-step approach will help.

**STEP ONE:** Think about your goal and make a note of five specific reasons why you want to achieve it. If you want to lose weight and feel more energetic, your reasons could be (1) so I'll feel more confident and comfortable in my body; (2) so I'll have more stamina to keep up with my kids; (3) so I can lead a fuller life; (4) so I will feel less exhausted at the end of the day; and (5) so I'll be willing to try new athletic endeavors.

**STEP TWO:** Imagine how it would feel to actually achieve that goal. Visualize a slimmer, more energetic you. How would you feel? How would you move? What would you be able to do that you can't do now? How much would you enjoy that? By picturing the fruits of your efforts, you'll become much more committed to pursuing your goal.

**STEP THREE:** Give yourself tools to help you get to your goal when your motivation wanes. Here are three strategies to help you go the distance:

**IDENTIFY INSPIRING MENTORS:** Scan your surroundings for people whose energy and enthusiasm you truly admire. Try to notice what they do to fuel their zest for life and talk to them about their secrets of leading an exuberant life Then, borrow and adapt their strategies so that they suit your life, and think of these people when you need a shot of motivation.

**EMBRACE AN ENERGIZING MANTRA:** Come up with a phrase or sentence that describes how you'd like to feel—perhaps something like "Nothing can stop me" or "I've got energy to burn"—and repeat it silently to yourself when you need a reminder that you have the will and the way to succeed. If this sounds like a form of positive self-talk, that's because it is. And it can help you kick-start the get-up-and-go you need to keep striving for your goal.

**OFFER YOURSELF REWARDS:** Each time you reach a milestone in your goal—whether it's losing five pounds or walking an additional mile—reward yourself with a treat for moving in the right direction. Draw up a wish list of small indulgences—a manicure, a bouquet of flowers, or a new CD, for example—for just this purpose, and keep it in a handy spot.

# Living Mindfully

Living a life that's abundant in energy and personal satisfaction requires living with intention. Many of us muddle our way through the days, weeks, and months of our lives without really thinking about what we want or treasure. In order to feel truly connected to your life, it helps to have a sense of purpose—or mission—that guides you in your actions. What's your personal vision? What values drive you in your life? Do you have a dream that's near and dear to your heart? What core beliefs do you embrace about what it means to be a valuable person? Answering these questions with full honesty can help you define what's important to you and discover an unrealized sense of intention or purpose in your life.

Having a sense of purpose also can bring enormous clarity to your life, which can, in turn, have an energy-boosting effect. What's more, research has found that having a sense of meaning in your life is an essential ingredient in personal happiness. In a recent study involving 347 people, a researcher at Middle Tennessee State University found that meaningfulness was a more powerful predictor of subjective well-being (aka happiness) than self-esteem, positive social relationships, and optimism.

When you are guided by a sense of meaning or purpose, chances are your life will begin to seem more manageable and better integrated. Everyday decision making becomes much easier, for example, if you make mindful choices that are in sync with your sense of purpose. After all, being mindful means living in the present, not the past or the future. It means keeping an eye on what's most precious to you. It means living with a sense of awareness of your own actions and how they relate to the reality and direction of your life. It means becoming more cognizant of the little things you do on a daily basis and whether these actions will help you or hinder you as you pursue your goals. When you live in harmony with these elements, you are living consciously, which can make it easier to separate the wheat from the chaff and guide your life, your career, or your relationships in a direction that will improve their quality. And these improvements can, in turn, help you reclaim your fervor for life. As Jon Kabat-Zinn, Ph.D., founder of the Stress Reduction Clinic at the University of Massachusetts Medical Center, puts it, "Mindfulness provides a simple but powerful route for getting ourselves unstuck, back into touch with our own wisdom and vitality."

Cultivating a sense of mindfulness—along with a proactive approach that enables you to take action that's in line with your goals and values—can help you get back in tune with your inherent vitality. After all, when you are mindful enough of your actions that you don't constantly misplace your keys or have to search for important papers on your cluttered desk, you'll be able to direct that unspent energy toward activities that will bring you closer to your goals. Plus, when you engage in each moment, you'll experience life more fully, and this can replenish your energy again and again. And when you stop worrying about all the "what ifs" and start addressing the positive prospects in your life, you'll probably rediscover psychological and emotional resources you'd forgotten you had. Indeed, the more open and receptive you are to the possibilities of life, the more nourishment you'll be providing to your body, mind, and spirit.

# Enhancing Your Energy Flow

As you know by now, it's all a matter of balance when it comes to turning an energy breakdown into an energy breakthrough. The goal is to strike a balance between the energy you expend and the energy you need to replenish, and to achieve balance among your physical, emotional, and spiritual well-being. Aiming toward this goal can help you gain a steadier flow of energy in your life, although it's important to remind yourself that no one's energy is perfectly balanced 365 days a year. Undoubtedly, you'll feel more vim and vigor on some days than others, but when you do feel enervated on an ongoing basis, view your fatigue as a signal that something in your body, your mind, or your life requires attention and perhaps a bit of retooling. What matters most is that you listen to the message your body is sending you—and that you try to do something to remedy the feeling.

What will solve one person's energy shortage may be quite different from what will do the trick for another person. There isn't a one-size-fits-all cure for energy crises. For some people, improving their eating habits and losing weight may prove to be the answer. For others, getting into shape and making exercise a habit could be the ticket to a more energetic life. And for still others, improving the quality of their slumber or finding new ways to relieve stress could be just what they need to recapture their zest for life. The only way to give yourself a personal energy makeover is to pinpoint the factors that are likely robbing you of energy, then to start taking better care of yourself by trying measures that are appropriate for those culprits.

While you're introducing some of the long-term solutions for your flagging energy, you can also use some of the strategies described in Chapter 6, which are likely to boost your energy more immediately. This combination of longer-acting and more instant measures will help you continue on your quest for more energy. It will also help you stay focused on what's happening here and now, rather than somewhere else or some other time. After all, what's likely to bolster your energy more than anything else is making your health and well-being a priority in your life and taking the time to restore your batteries on a regular basis. Just as you would advise your children, your spouse, or other loved ones to rest or relax when they need to and to engage in activities they truly enjoy (and to skip those they don't whenever possible), you should apply the same good advice to yourself.

This is *your* life—shouldn't you enjoy it as much as you can? If you take steps to nurture your energy, your energy will return the favor exponentially. After all, the care and feeding of your personal energy will help you feel better as well as be in better health. It will help you lead a more meaningful existence and function more efficiently with less stress and strain. It's a way to become more active as well as calmer, and to reclaim a youthful enthusiasm that's coupled with the wisdom of experience. Reclaiming your lost energy is really the most thoughtful gift you could give to yourself and those you love. After all, when you become happier, healthier, livelier, and more energetic, you will be making the world an even brighter place.

# PART 2

# Fueling Your Energy

# 8

## Four Weeks to Better Eating

### Day 1 ≡

**BREAKFAST (5 POINTS)**

3/4 c. raisin bran cereal with 1/2 c. fat-free milk (2)

1 c. orange juice (2)

1 c. coffee with 1/2 c. steamed fat-free milk (1)

**LUNCH (6 POINTS)**

White Bean Dip* (2)

1 large (2 oz.) whole-wheat pita (2)

Spinach Salad

*Toss 1 c. baby spinach and 1 c. sliced mushrooms with 1 tsp. each balsamic vinegar and olive oil; season with salt and pepper to taste. (1)*

1 kiwi fruit (1)

Unsweetened iced tea (0)

**DINNER (9 POINTS)**

Broiled Beef Strip Steak with Garlic Mashed Potatoes

*Marinate beef strip steak (5–6 oz.) in 2 tbsp. fat-free Italian dressing mixed with 1 tsp. honey mustard and 1/2 tsp. coarsely ground black pepper for 30 minutes. Meanwhile, peel, quarter, and boil 1 medium potato with 2 peeled whole garlic cloves in lightly salted water until tender, about 20 minutes. Drain and mash together with 2 tbsp. half-and-half. Remove strip steak from marinade (discard excess marinade) and broil about 5 minutes per side, for medium-rare. (8)*

1 c. steamed green beans (0)

1 c. baby carrots with 1/2 tsp. chopped fresh dill (1)

*Recipe on page 175.*

1 c. fat-free sugar-free vanilla pudding made with fat-free milk, topped with 3
   tbsp. toasted wheat germ (4)

1 banana (2)

**TOTAL DAILY POINTS: 26**

## Day 2

**BREAKFAST (6.5 POINTS)**

1 whole-wheat English muffin (2)

1 tsp. almond butter (1)

1$^1$/2 tbsp. spreadable fruit (1)

1 c. light vanilla yogurt with $^1$/2 c. frozen unsweetened cherries (2.5)

**LUNCH (7 POINTS)**

Veggie and Egg Salad

*On a bed of 1 c. baby spinach leaves, arrange 1 c. sliced cooked beets, 1 sliced
hard-cooked egg, and $^1$/4 c. garbanzo beans. Top with 2 tbsp. light sour cream mixed
with 1 tbsp. fat-free milk and 1 tsp. horseradish. Sprinkle with 1 tsp. sunflower
seeds. (4)*

$^3$/4 oz. thin bread sticks (2)

1 small apple, sliced (1)

**DINNER (6.5 POINTS)**

Roasted Chicken and Vegetables

*Combine 1 tbsp. each Dijon mustard and light mayonnaise with 1 tsp. sunflower oil.
Brush over 4 oz. boneless, skinless chicken breast, 1 quartered sweet onion, 1 quartered small potato (skin on), and 4 large mushrooms, all placed in a nonstick baking
pan in a single layer. Bake, uncovered, at 350° F, about 30 minutes, or until chicken
juices run clear and potato is tender. (6.5)*

1 c. red and green pepper strips (0)

Unsweetened iced tea (0)

**SNACKS (3 POINTS)**

Strawberry Smoothie

*Purée 1 1/2 c. frozen unsweetened strawberries with 1 c. fat-free buttermilk in a blender. (3)*

1 c. sliced radishes drizzled with 1 tsp. fat-free ranch dressing (0)

**TOTAL DAILY POINTS: 23**

## Day 3

### BREAKFAST (5 POINTS)

1 1/2 c. bran flakes cereal (2)

1 c. fat-free milk (2)

1 c. fresh pineapple chunks (1)

### LUNCH (9 POINTS)

1 fast-food hamburger (6)

1 side salad with 2 tbsp. reduced-calorie dressing (2)

1 c. baby carrots (1)

Seltzer with a lemon wedge (0)

### DINNER (8 POINTS)

Simple Vegetable-Pasta Sauté

*Heat 1 1/2 tsp. sunflower oil in a nonstick pan. Sauté 1 medium onion, sliced, and 1 crushed garlic clove for 3–5 minutes. Add 1 1/2 c. chopped kale and a dash of crushed red pepper; cook, covered, until kale is tender, about 5 minutes. Add 1 c. cooked bowtie pasta and heat through. Top with 1 1/2 tbsp. of grated Parmesan cheese. (7)*

1 sliced tomato, seasoned with dried oregano, salt, and pepper to taste (0)

2 purple plums (1)

### SNACKS (2 POINTS)

Iced Mocha Coffee

*Whisk together 1/2 c. cold coffee, 1 tsp. unsweetened cocoa powder, and 1/2 c. fat-free milk. Serve over ice. (1)*

1 c. raw zucchini and red pepper strips with 1 tbsp. reduced-calorie, cracked-pepper salad dressing (1)

**TOTAL DAILY POINTS: 24**

# Day 4 ≡

**BREAKFAST (5 POINTS)**

1 c. cooked oatmeal with $1/2$ c. fat-free milk (3)

1 small apple, chopped (1)

3 toasted walnut halves, chopped (1)

**LUNCH (7 POINTS)**

Ham-and-Swiss Sandwich

*Spread 2 tsp. honey mustard over 2 slices high-fiber, whole-wheat bread. Layer 2 lettuce leaves, 2 thin slices purple onion, 1 slice tomato, 1 oz. lean ham, and 1 oz. Swiss cheese between the bread slices. (6)*

1 yellow pepper cut into strips (0)

1 dill pickle (0)

2 purple plums (1)

**DINNER (11 POINTS)**

Braised Chicken with Lentils and Gremolata* (10)

1 c. steamed broccoli, tossed with 1 tsp. lemon juice and 1 drop of chili oil (0)

1 c. low-salt mixed vegetable juice (1)

**SNACK (4 POINTS)**

Creamy Orange Shake

*Whisk together 1 c. light vanilla yogurt with $1/2$ c. orange juice and 2 drops vanilla extract. (3)*

2 ginger snaps (1)

**TOTAL DAILY POINTS: 27**

*Recipe on page 194.

# Day 5 ≣

## BREAKFAST (5 POINTS)

1 c. mini shredded wheat cereal (2)

1 c. blueberries (1)

1 c. fat-free milk (2)

## LUNCH (7 POINTS)

Black Bean Tortilla Wrap

*Spread 2 Tbsp. fat-free black bean dip, 1 diced plum tomato, and 4 Tbsp. shredded pepper-jack cheese onto a 10-inch whole-wheat flour tortilla. Microwave on high for 1 minute, until cheese starts to melt. Add 1 c. shredded romaine lettuce and 2 tbsp. salsa, and fold wrap together.* (7)

1 c. jicama sticks (0)

Unsweetened herbal iced tea with lemon (0)

## DINNER (12 POINTS)

Grilled Red Snapper Fillet

*Brush 6 oz. red snapper fillet with 1/2 tsp. sunflower oil and broil until opaque, about 7 minutes. Sprinkle with 1 tsp. lemon juice, 2 tsp. chopped chives, and a dash of black pepper.* (4.5)

1 c. steamed spinach (0)

1 c. cooked brown rice (cooked in chicken broth with 1/2 tsp. salt-free butter) (4.5)

1 small (4 oz.) glass white wine (2)

3 fresh apricots or 6 dried apricot halves (1)

## SNACK (2 POINTS)

3 c. light microwave-popped popcorn (1)

1/2 c. light yogurt topped with 1/4 c. chopped strawberries (1)

1 c. broccoli florets (0)

## TOTAL DAILY POINTS: 26

# Day 6 ≡

## BREAKFAST (6 POINTS)

1 (4-inch) low-fat toaster waffle (2)

1 tbsp. maple syrup (1)

$^1/_2$ c. sliced peaches (1)

1 c. fat-free milk (2)

## LUNCH (10 POINTS)

Pasta Salad Tonnato* (5)

1 ($^3/_4$ oz.) crispbread (1)

1 c. blackberries (1)

1 c. fat-free sugar-free lemon pudding made with fat-free milk (3)

## DINNER (9.5 POINTS)

Grilled Pork Kebabs

*Cube 4 oz. pork tenderloin and rub cubes with $^1/_8$ tsp. seasoned salt. Cut $^1/_2$ red and $^1/_2$ yellow pepper into 1-inch chunks; cut 1 small zucchini into 1-inch pieces. Thread 5 medium mushrooms with pork, peppers, and zucchini onto 2 skewers. Lightly brush kebabs with a mixture of 2 tbsp. apricot preserves thinned with 1 tsp. cider vinegar. Broil 6 minutes; turn and cook another 6 to 8 minutes, or until pork is cooked through.* (6.5)

$^1/_2$ c. cooked brown rice (2)

1 c. fresh pineapple chunks (1)

## SNACKS (1.5 POINTS)

Orange Juice Spritzer

*Pour $^1/_4$ c. orange juice and 1 c. berry-flavored carbonated water over 3–4 ice cubes; garnish with a slice of lemon.* (.5)

2 ginger snaps (1)

4 celery sticks and $^1/_2$ c. raw turnip slices, sprinkled with a dash of salt (0)

## TOTAL DAILY POINTS: 27

*Recipe on page 191.

# Day 7 ≣

**BREAKFAST (9 POINTS)**

Mexican Omelet
> *Heat a nonstick skillet sprayed with cooking spray over medium heat. Whisk 2 large eggs and pour into skillet; cook until just set. Top with 1 oz. shredded pepper-jack cheese, 2 tbsp. salsa, and 2 tbsp. chopped green chilis. Fold in half and continue cooking until cheese begins to melt.* (7)

1 slice whole-wheat toast (1)

$1/2$ c. grapefruit juice (1)

**LUNCH (6 POINTS)**

1 c. Weight Watchers Garden Vegetable Soup
> *Spray large saucepan with nonstick cooking spray; sauté $1/3$ c. sliced carrot, $1/4$ c. diced onion and 1 minced garlic clove over low heat, about 5 minutes. Add $1 1/2$ c. fat-free chicken, beef or vegetable broth, $3/4$ c. chopped green cabbage, $1/4$ c. green beans, $1/2$ tbsp. tomato paste, $1/4$ tsp. each dried basil and oregano, and a pinch of salt; bring to a boil. Lower heat and simmer, covered, about 15 minutes or until beans are tender. Stir in $1/4$ diced zucchini and heat through. Serve hot.* (0)

1 large (2 oz.) whole wheat pita with $1/4$ c. hummus (5)

1 celery stalk (0)

2 small clementines (1)

**DINNER (10 POINTS)**

Lemon Veal Chops with Tomato and Olive Couscous* (8)

1 c. steamed string beans with a dash of lemon pepper (0)

$1/2$ c. cubed papaya (.5)

$1/2$ c. fat-free sugar-free vanilla pudding made with fat-free milk (1.5)

**SNACKS (2 POINTS)**

1 c. red and yellow pepper strips (0)

> *Mix 1 c. Swiss-almond flavored coffee, 1 c. steamed fat-free milk, and 2 drops almond extract.* (2)

**TOTAL DAILY POINTS: 27**

*Recipe on page 214.

# Day 8 ≣

**BREAKFAST (5 POINTS)**

1½ c. bran flakes cereal (2)

1 c. fat-free milk (2)

1 c. sliced peaches (1)

**LUNCH (12 POINTS)**

Ham and Coleslaw Hoagie
*Mix ½ c. of shredded red cabbage with 2 tsp. each reduced-calorie mayonnaise and Dijon mustard. Cut open a 2 oz. hoagie bun and layer it with 2 oz. sliced lean deli ham, 1 oz. Swiss cheese, and the cabbage. (9)*

12 (1 oz.) baked tortilla chips (2)

1 pear (1)

**DINNER (7 POINTS)**

3 oz. smoked cooked trout (3)

2 small boiled potatoes with 3 tbsp. light sour cream mixed with 1 tbsp. horse-radish (3)

6 steamed asparagus spears with dash of fresh lemon juice (0)

1 c. sliced cucumber tossed with 1 tbsp. mixed fresh herbs such as chives, dill, and parsley (0)

2 purple plums (1)

**SNACKS (3 POINTS)**

1 c. blueberries mixed with ½ c. light lemon yogurt (2)

1 c. baby carrots (1)

**TOTAL DAILY POINTS: 27**

# Day 9 ≡

**BREAKFAST (5 POINTS)**

1 whole-wheat English muffin (2)

1 tbsp. orange marmalade (1)

$1^1/2$ c. sliced strawberries with 2 tbsp. fat-free half-and-half (2)

**LUNCH (11 POINTS)**

Cock-a-Leekie* (7)

2 slices (1 oz. each) toasted, high-fiber oat bran bread (2)

1 c. fat-free milk (2)

**DINNER (7 POINTS)**

Grilled Pork Chop with Peppery Corn

*Brush a 3 oz. boneless pork loin chop with 1 tbsp. barbecue sauce and grill in a nonstick grill pan about 5 minutes on each side, or until juices run clear. Meanwhile, sauté $1/2$ sliced red pepper and $1/2$ diced jalapeño pepper in 1 tsp. sunflower oil. When peppers begin to brown, stir in $1/2$ c. whole-kernel corn and heat through.* (5)

Citrus Salad

*Toss 1 c. chopped romaine lettuce with 2 thin slices of purple onion, $1/2$ c. fresh grapefruit sections, and 1 tsp. each balsamic vinegar and sunflower oil. Season to taste with salt and pepper.* (2)

Unsweetened iced tea (0)

**SNACKS (4 POINTS)**

Orange and Buttermilk Smoothie

*Blend 1 c. fat-free buttermilk with $1/4$ c. orange sherbet and $1/2$ tsp. orange zest.* (3)

1 c. cubed honeydew melon (1)

**TOTAL DAILY POINTS: 27**

*Recipe on page 180.

# Day 10 ≣

**BREAKFAST (6 POINTS)**

Lemon-Cheesecake Waffle

*Toast 1 (1 oz.) frozen Belgian waffle. Meanwhile, mix ¹/2 c. fat-free ricotta cheese, 2 tbsp. raisins, ¹/4 tsp. lemon zest, and 1 tbsp. half-and-half; spread over toasted waffle. Microwave on high until hot, about 30 seconds. Sprinkle with ¹/2 tsp. powdered sugar.* (5.5)

¹/2 small grapefruit (.5)

**LUNCH (9 POINTS)**

1 small fast-food hamburger with ketchup, lettuce, onion, mustard, and dill pickle (6)

1 c. fat-free milk (2)

1 small apple (1)

**DINNER (11 POINTS)**

1 c. bean and lentil stew (6)

1 c. cooked brown rice (4)

¹/2 c. vegetable raita with 1 tbsp. chopped mint (1)

1 c. sparkling mineral water (0)

**SNACKS (1 POINT)**

1 c. cubed watermelon (1)

1 c. jicama sticks (0)

**TOTAL DAILY POINTS: 27**

# Day 11 ≡

**BREAKFAST (5 POINTS)**

1 c. cooked oatmeal with $^1/_2$ c. fat-free milk (3)

2 tbsp. dried cherries (1)

1 c. coffee with $^1/_2$ c. steamed fat-free milk, dusted with $^1/_2$ tsp. cocoa powder (1)

**LUNCH (8.5 POINTS)**

Chicken-Edamame Salad in a Pita

*Cube 2 oz. of cooked boneless skinless chicken breast and combine with $^1/_4$ c. each cooked edamame (fresh, green soy beans) and diced celery, 4 tsp. each reduced-calorie mayonnaise and sliced green onion, and 1 tsp. sweet pickle relish. Season to taste with a dash of salt and cayenne pepper. Serve in 1 small (1 oz.) whole-wheat pita pocket. (6.5)*

1 c. baby carrots (1)

1 c. grapes (1)

**DINNER (9 POINTS)**

1 c. angel hair pasta with $^1/_2$ c. store-bought pasta sauce (6)

Tuscan Beans

*In a small nonstick skillet, heat $^1/_2$ tsp. olive oil. Add 3 fresh sage leaves, cut into slivers, and cook for 30 seconds. Add $^1/_2$ c. canned, drained white beans, and $^1/_8$ tsp. each salt and freshly ground pepper, and heat through. (2.5)*

Spinach Salad

*In a small bowl, mash 2 cloves roasted garlic. Mix with $^1/_2$ tsp. olive oil; slowly add 1 tbsp. fat-free Italian dressing. Toss with 1 c. baby spinach; garnish with a slice of roasted red pepper. (0.5)*

**SNACKS (5.5 POINTS)**

Fruited-Honey Yogurt

*Whisk 1 c. plain fat-free yogurt, 1 tbsp. warmed honey, and $^1/_2$ tsp. lemon zest until honey is dissolved. Stir in 1 c. blueberries. (5)*

$^1/_2$ c. snow peas and $^1/_2$ c. raw turnip sticks with 1 tbsp. fat-free ranch dressing (.5)

**TOTAL DAILY POINTS: 28**

# Day 12 ≡

**BREAKFAST (5 POINTS)**

1 c. light vanilla yogurt with 1 1/2 c. raspberries (3)

1 small (2 oz.) fat-free, store-bought bran muffin (2)

Coffee or tea (0)

**LUNCH (9.5 POINTS)**

Orzo-Surimi Salad

*Mix 1 c. cooked orzo pasta with 1/4 c. cooked green peas, 1/2 c. shredded surimi, 1 tbsp. each reduced-fat mayonnaise, chili sauce, and chives, 2 tsp. lemon juice, 1/8 tsp. lemon zest, and a sprinkle of chopped fresh dill. Serve on a bed of 1 1/2 c. shredded red leaf lettuce and 1 sliced tomato. (7.5)*

1 c. fat-free milk (2)

**DINNER (7.5 POINTS)**

Curried Turkey Cutlets* (4)

1/2 c. cooked brown rice (2)

1 c. steamed cauliflower florets tossed with 1/2 tsp. butter (.5)

1 c. salad greens and 1/4 c. chopped cucumber tossed with 1 tsp. each rice wine vinegar and sunflower oil (1)

**SNACKS (2 POINTS)**

3 c. light microwave-popped popcorn (1)

1 pear (1)

**TOTAL DAILY POINTS: 24**

*Recipe on page 202.*

# Day 13 ☰

## BREAKFAST (9 POINTS)

2-Egg Scramble
> *Heat 1 tsp. sunflower oil in a nonstick skillet. Whisk 2 large eggs with 1 tbsp. fat-free milk, and salt and pepper to taste. Cook until eggs are set; top with 1 tbsp. grated cheddar cheese and heat through until cheese melts. Serve with 2 tbsp. salsa.* (6)

2 slices (2 oz.) high-fiber, whole-wheat bread, toasted (2)

1 orange (1)

## LUNCH (5 POINTS)

1 c. canned gazpacho (1)

3 whole-wheat soda crackers (1)

1 c. each zucchini slices and red pepper rings with $^{1}/_{2}$ c. fat-free bean dip (1)

1 c. fat-free milk (2)

## DINNER (8 POINTS)

Caramelized Sweet-Onion Pizza
> *Preheat oven to 400° F. Heat 1 tsp. oil in a nonstick skillet. Add 1 sliced sweet onion and cook until browned. Meanwhile, split a 2 oz. whole-wheat pita and place both halves on a baking sheet. Distribute the onion evenly over both halves, then top each half with $^{1}/_{2}$ oz. crumbled blue cheese. Bake for 5 minutes or until heated through.* (6)

1 c. chopped romaine lettuce topped with 1 chopped tomato and 2 tbsp. fat-free Italian dressing (0)

1 (12 oz.) light beer (2)

## SNACKS (4 POINTS)

Vanilla Latte
> *Mix 1 c. vanilla-flavored coffee with $^{1}/_{2}$ c. fat-free steamed milk.* (1)

Power Parfait
> *Layer $^{1}/_{2}$ c. light lime yogurt with $^{1}/_{2}$ c. sliced strawberries, $^{1}/_{2}$ chopped kiwi fruit, and 3 tbsp. wheat germ in a wineglass; top with 1 tsp. brown sugar.* (3)

## TOTAL DAILY POINTS: 26

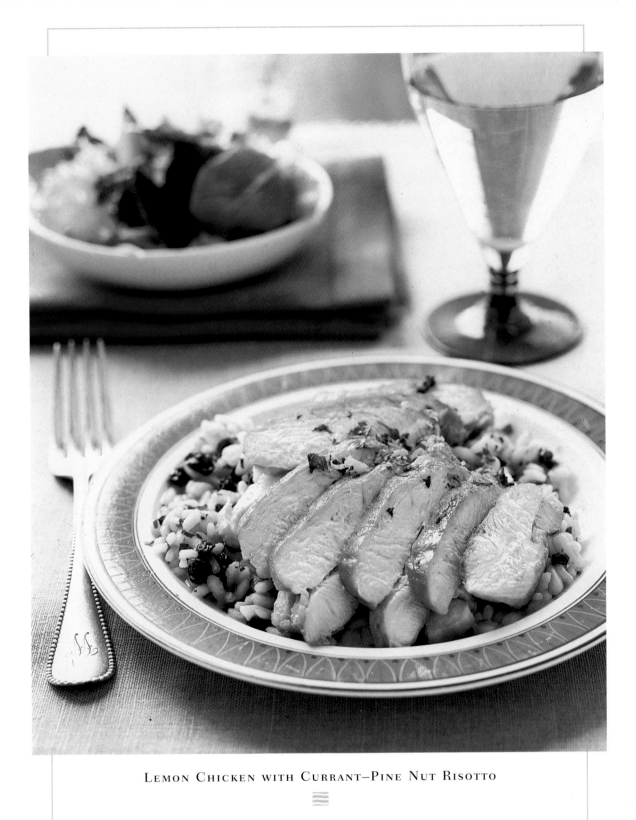

LEMON CHICKEN WITH CURRANT–PINE NUT RISOTTO

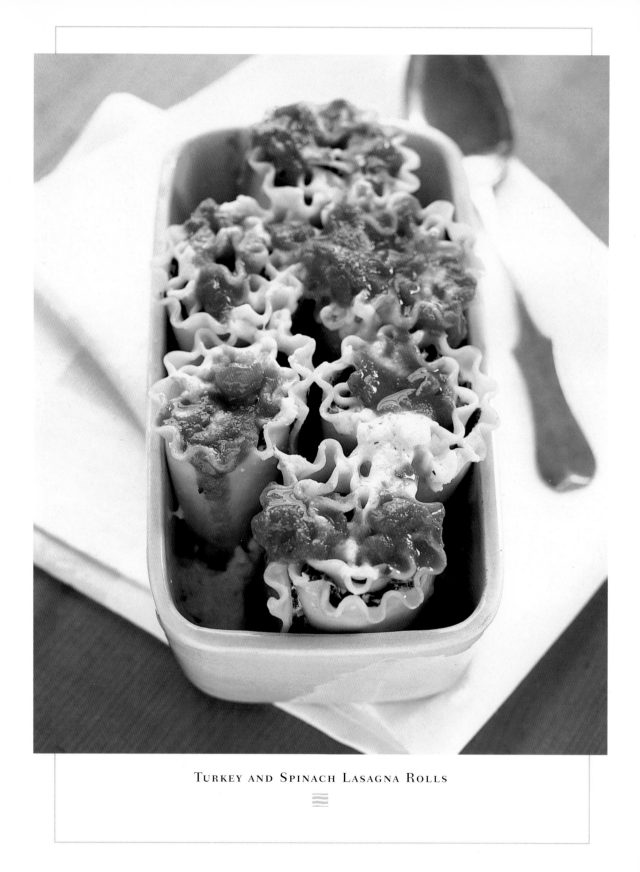

TURKEY AND SPINACH LASAGNA ROLLS

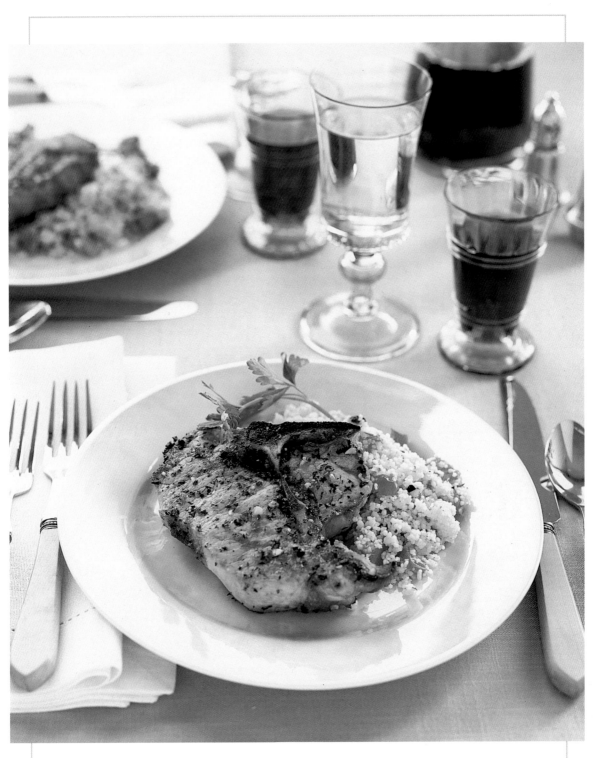

LEMON VEAL CHOPS WITH TOMATO AND OLIVE COUSCOUS

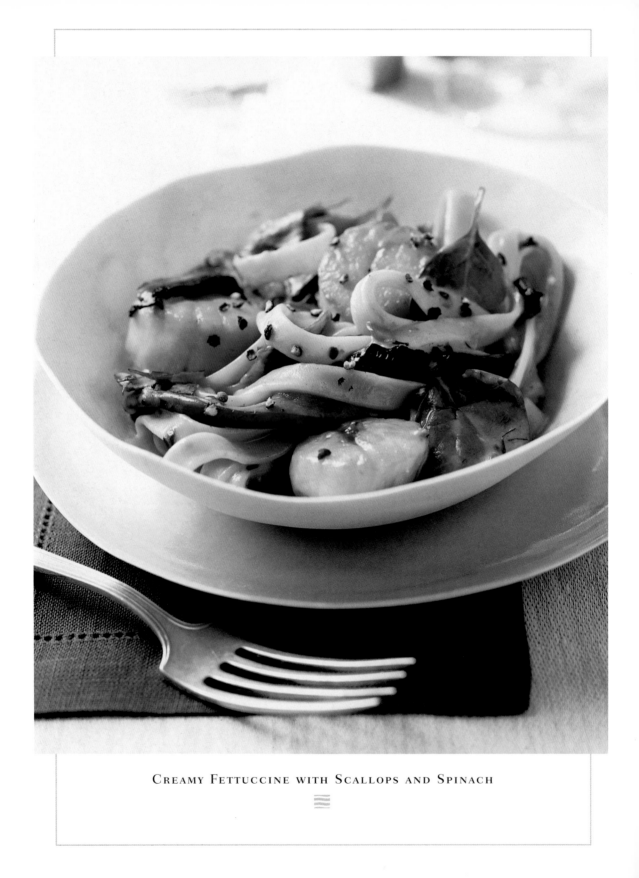

CREAMY FETTUCCINE WITH SCALLOPS AND SPINACH

# Day 14 ≡

## BREAKFAST (7 POINTS)

1 small (2 oz.) whole-wheat bagel, toasted (3)

2 tbsp. light cream cheese (1)

1/2 c. mango slices (1)

Cinnamon Steamer
*Microwave 1 c. fat-free milk on high for 1 minute in a large mug. Whisk in 1 tsp. of honey and 1/4 tsp. of cinnamon until milk is frothy and cinnamon is dissolved. (2)*

## LUNCH (7 POINTS)

Shrimp, Fennel, and Grapes in Cantaloupe Halves* (6)

6 melba toast rounds (1)

1/2 c. low-salt mixed vegetable juice (0)

## DINNER (10 POINTS)

Poached Salmon
*Heat 1/4 c. dry vermouth with 3 lemon slices, 3 sprigs parsley, and 1 small sliced scallion in a saucepan over medium heat. Add a 4 oz. salmon fillet and simmer for 5–8 minutes, turning once, until salmon becomes opaque. (6)*

2 small potatoes, boiled (2)

1 c. cucumber slices topped with 2 tbsp. light plain yogurt mixed with 1/8 tsp. chopped garlic, 1 tsp. chopped fresh mint, and a dash of cayenne (0)

1 c. mixed berries sprinkled with 1 tbsp. Grand Marnier (2)

## SNACKS (3 POINTS)

1 c. fat-free sugar-free chocolate pudding made with fat-free milk (3)

1 c. steamed broccoli and cauliflower florets marinated in 1 tbsp. fat-free Italian dressing (0)

## TOTAL DAILY POINTS: 27

*Recipe on page 189.

# Day 15 ≡

**BREAKFAST** ( 6 POINTS )

Peach-Crunch Parfait
*Layer 8 oz. light vanilla yogurt, 1 cubed medium peach, 5 tbsp. low-fat granola cereal, and 3 tbsp. toasted wheat germ in a 12 oz. glass. (6)*
Coffee or tea (0)

**LUNCH** ( 10.5 POINTS )

Palm Springs Tuna Pocket
*Fill a large (2 oz.) whole-wheat pita with $^1/_2$ c. each bean sprouts and shredded carrot. Stuff with $^1/_2$ c. drained water-packed tuna mixed with 2 tsp. reduced-calorie mayonnaise and 1 tsp. each diced red onion and finely chopped dill. (6.5)*
1 c. cubed mango (2)
1 c. fat-free milk (2)

**DINNER** ( 8.5 POINTS )

Sesame Noodles and Vegetables
*Heat 1 c. cooked linguine, $^1/_2$ c. steamed broccoli florets, and $^1/_2$ c. each snow peas and thinly sliced red pepper strips in a nonstick skillet with 1 tsp. each sunflower and sesame oil. Remove from heat and sprinkle with 1 tsp. sesame seeds and a dash of crushed red pepper; toss. (6)*
1 small (4 oz.) glass white wine (2)
$^1/_2$ c. watermelon cubes (.5)

**SNACKS** ( 2 POINTS )

1 c. sliced cucumber with 1 tbsp. onion–sour cream dip thinned with 1 tbsp. fat-free milk (1)
3 c. light microwave-popped popcorn (1)

**TOTAL DAILY POINTS: 27**

# Day 16  ≋

**BREAKFAST (5 POINTS)**

3/4 c. bran flakes cereal (1)

1 banana (2)

1 c. fat-free milk (2)

**LUNCH (7 POINTS)**

Stuffed Sweet Potato

*Top a large, cooked sweet potato with 1/3 c. nonfat cottage cheese; sprinkle with 7 chopped walnut halves. (6.5)*

1 c. steamed broccoli florets with 1/2 tsp. sunflower oil and a dash of cayenne (0.5)

Unsweetened iced tea (0)

**DINNER (10 POINTS)**

California Cheese Burger

*Combine 4 oz. lean ground beef and 2 tbsp. low-fat shredded cheddar cheese. Shape into a patty and broil until cooked through, and juices run clear, about 10 minutes. Serve on a light hamburger bun with 1 small tomato, sliced, and 2 lettuce leaves. (9)*

1 c. steamed zucchini sprinkled with 1/2 tsp. dried basil and a dash of lemon pepper (0)

1 c. ripe guava chunks (1)

**SNACKS (5 POINTS)**

1/2 c. hazelnut coffee with 1 c. fat-free steamed milk (2)

Blueberry Clafouti* (3)

**TOTAL DAILY POINTS: 27**

*Recipe on page 242.

# Day 17 ≣

**BREAKFAST (9 POINTS)**

Tomato-Egg Melt

*Heat 1 tsp. sunflower oil in a medium nonstick skillet. Whisk together 1 egg white, 1 whole egg, and 1/4 c. shredded part-skim mozzarella cheese. Pour egg mixture into skillet and cook until firm. Spoon onto 1/2 large bagel and top with 1 tomato slice.* (8)

1 c. honeydew melon cubes (1)

Coffee or tea (0)

**LUNCH (6 POINTS)**

Easy Three-Bean Salad

*Toss 1/4 c. canned, drained black beans and 1/2 c. canned, drained red kidney beans with 1 c. steamed green beans; drizzle with 1 tsp. each sunflower oil and red wine vinegar. Sprinkle with a pinch each of dried oregano and garlic powder.* (3)

1 large (2 oz.) whole-wheat pita, toasted and cut into wedges (2)

2 small purple plums (1)

**DINNER (8 POINTS)**

Summer Harvest Risotto

*Combine 1/4 c. arborio rice and 2 tbsp. chicken broth in a medium saucepan placed over medium heat. Continue adding more broth, 2 tbsp. at a time, as previous addition is absorbed. Simmer until rice is cooked through, about 15 minutes. Stir in 1/2 c. each chopped yellow squash and scallions, and 1 tsp. minced garlic. Top with 2 tbsp. grated Parmesan cheese.* (6)

1 c. baby field greens with 2 tbsp. fat-free Italian dressing (0)

1 c. fat-free milk (2)

**SNACKS (3 POINTS)**

Berry Delight

*Combine 3/4 c. each sliced strawberries and raspberries with 1 c. fat-free milk and 3 ice cubes in a blender.* (3)

1 c. snow peas (0)

**TOTAL DAILY POINTS: 26**

# Day 18 ☰

**BREAKFAST (5 POINTS)**

1 1/2 c. bran flakes cereal (2)
1 c. cubed papaya (1)
1 c. fat-free milk (2)
Coffee or tea (0)

**LUNCH (8 POINTS)**

Pepper-Jack Quesadilla
*Layer 1/4 cup shredded Monterey Jack cheese and 1 sliced roasted red pepper be-tween two 6-inch corn tortillas. Heat in a nonstick skillet until cheese begins to melt, about 3 minutes; turn and heat through.* (5)

Chopped Salad
*Combine 1/2 c. each chopped tomato and cucumber; toss with 2 tsp. lemon juice and 1 tsp. olive oil.* (1)

1 c. fat-free milk (2)

**DINNER (9 POINTS)**

Herbed Halibut
*Coat an 8 oz. halibut fillet with 2 tbsp. fresh lemon juice and 1 tsp. sunflower oil. Sprinkle with 1 tsp. each chopped parsley, oregano, and dill; bake at 350° F. until fish turns opaque, about 10 minutes.* (6)

1 c. steamed spinach sprinkled with 1 tbsp. toasted pine nuts (1)
1/2 c. cooked brown rice (2)
Raspberry seltzer (0)

**SNACKS (1 POINT)**

1 c. fresh pineapple cubes (1)
1/2 c. mixed vegetable juice spiced with 3 drops hot sauce and heated with 1/2 c. beef bouillion (0)

**TOTAL DAILY POINTS: 23**

# Day 19 ☰

**BREAKFAST** (7 POINTS)

Banana Maple Toast
*Whisk together ¹/₄ c. fat-free egg substitute, 1 tbsp. fat-free milk, ¹/₈ tsp. vanilla extract, and a pinch of cinnamon; dip 2 slices whole-wheat bread into mixture and sprinkle with 3 tbsp. wheat germ. Cook bread slices in a nonstick skillet, turning once, for about 3 minutes. Top with 1 sliced banana and 1 tbsp. maple syrup.* (7)

Coffee or tea (0)

**LUNCH** (7 POINTS)

Peanut Butter and Honey Sandwich
*Between 2 slices reduced-calorie whole-wheat bread, spread 1 tbsp. peanut butter and 1 tbsp. honey.* (4)

¹/₂ c. celery sticks (0)

1 c. fat-free milk (2)

1 pear (1)

**DINNER** (7 POINTS)

Orange Beef with Noodles* (4)

Garlic Bok Choy
*In a nonstick skillet, heat 1 tsp. sunflower oil and 1 minced garlic clove, a pinch of crushed red pepper, and ¹/₂ tsp. reduced-sodium soy sauce. Add 2 c. chopped bok choy and sauté until just wilted.* (1)

¹/₂ c. pineapple sorbet (2)

Unsweetened iced lemon tea (0)

**SNACKS** (4 POINTS)

Yogurt Freeze
*Combine 1 c. light vanilla yogurt with 1 c. blueberries or frozen peaches in a blender; serve immediately.* (3)

1 kiwi fruit (1)

**TOTAL DAILY POINTS: 25**

*Recipe on page 211.

# Day 20 ≣

**BREAKFAST** (6 POINTS)

3/4 c. raisin bran cereal (1)

1 c. fat-free milk (2)

6 canned, water-packed apricot halves (1)

Dutch Hot Chocolate

*In a small saucepan, heat 1 c. fat-free milk with 1 tsp. unsweetened cocoa powder, 1/4 tsp. cinnamon, and a pinch of cloves. Whisk until spices are blended in and milk is frothy on top.* (2)

**LUNCH** (9 POINTS)

Smoked Salmon Wrap

*Combine 4 tbsp. nonfat cream cheese and 1 tbsp. chopped dill; divide between two 6-inch whole-wheat flour tortillas. Layer 1 oz. smoked salmon, 2 cooked asparagus spears, and 1 tbsp. minced sweet onion onto each; roll and secure with a toothpick.* (7)

1 c. mixed greens with 1 tbsp. fat-free Italian dressing (0)

2 c. frozen seedless red grapes (2)

**DINNER** (5 POINTS)

Baked Scallops

*Combine 1 tsp. each lemon juice and melted salt-free butter, 1 tbsp. white wine and a pinch of dried thyme; pour over 1/2 c. scallops and marinate 20 minutes. Bake in a small casserole dish in 450° F oven for 5 minutes.* (2)

1 steamed artichoke (0)

Lemonberry Shake

*In a blender, combine 1/2 c. light lemon yogurt with 1/3 c. fat-free milk, 1 c. blueberries, and 3 ice cubes.* (3)

**SNACKS** (4 POINTS)

3 c. light microwave-popped popcorn (1)

1 oz. beef jerky (3)

**TOTAL DAILY** POINTS: 24

# Day 21 ≣

**BREAKFAST (7 POINTS)**

Strawberries and Cream Bagel
*Top 1/2 whole-wheat bagel with 1 tbsp. cream cheese and 1 1/2 tbsp. strawberry spreadable fruit.* (5)

1 c. light strawberry yogurt (2)

Coffee or tea (0)

**LUNCH (7 POINTS)**

1 vegetarian burger (2)

1 light hamburger roll (2)

1 slice low-fat American cheese (2)

1/2 c. each shredded lettuce, chopped tomato, and onion (0)

1 c. carrot and celery sticks (0)

1 nectarine (1)

**DINNER (9 POINTS)**

Flounder en Papillote* (3)

1 large (8 oz.) baked potato (skin on) with 2 tbsp. light sour cream (4)

1 c. green and yellow squash slices and 1 c. red and green pepper strips sautéed in 1 tsp. olive oil (1)

1 kiwi fruit (1)

**SNACKS (2 POINTS)**

1 c. Weight Watchers Garden Vegetable Soup (see recipe, page 138) (0)

1 c. fat-free milk (2)

**TOTAL DAILY POINTS: 25**

*Recipe on page 226.

# Day 22 ≡

## BREAKFAST (8 POINTS)

1 large store-bought fat-free raisin bran muffin with 1 tbsp. blackberry spreadable fruit (5)

1 c. mixed berries (1)

1 c. fat-free milk (2)

## LUNCH (6 POINTS)

Honey-Dijon Chicken Sandwich
*Combine 1 tsp. each honey and Dijon mustard; spread onto 2 slices reduced-calorie whole-wheat bread and top with 2 tsp. reduced-calorie mayonnaise. Top with 3 oz. cooked boneless skinless chicken breast, 2 slices each red onion and tomato, and 1/4 c. alfalfa sprouts. (5)*

1 c. baby carrots (1)

Unsweetened iced tea (0)

## DINNER (9 POINTS)

Baked Ziti
*Combine 1 c. cooked ziti, 1/2 c. each tomato sauce and sliced yellow squash, and 1 tsp. olive oil. Spread in small casserole dish; top with 1/3 c. nonfat ricotta cheese and 1/4 c. shredded part-skim mozzarella cheese. Bake at 350° F. until heated through, about 15 minutes. (8)*

Crunchy Zucchini Sticks* (1)

1 c. arugula and lettuce leaves with 2 tbsp. fat-free Italian dressing (0)

## SNACKS (3 POINTS)

Creamy Cappuccino Freeze
*In a blender, combine 1/2 c. light vanilla yogurt, 1/2 c. fat-free milk, 1/4 c. brewed espresso, 3 ice cubes, 1/2 tsp. superfine sugar, and 1/4 tsp. cinnamon. (2)*

1 orange (1)

## TOTAL DAILY POINTS: 26

*Recipe on page 257.*

# Day 23 ≡

**BREAKFAST** (5 POINTS)

1 hard-cooked egg with salt and pepper to taste (2)

1 tomato, chopped (0)

2 slices high-fiber whole-wheat toast with 1 tsp. salt-free butter (3)

Coffee or tea (0)

**LUNCH** (9 POINTS)

Turkey Club Sandwich

*Toast 3 slices (3 oz.) high-fiber whole-wheat bread. Layer 1 slice with 2 slices (2 oz.) cooked skinless turkey breast, 2 lettuce leaves, 3 tomato slices, and 2 tsp. reduced-calorie mayonnaise. Top with another toast slice; layer with 1/4 c. shredded carrot, 4 cucumber slices, and 1 tsp. Dijon mustard. Top with remaining bread slice.* (6)

1 c. fat-free milk (2)

1 c. cantaloupe chunks (1)

**DINNER** (7 POINTS)

Tofu-Veggie Stir-Fry

*Stir-fry 1/3 c. cubed firm tofu and 1/2 c. each chopped mushrooms, bell peppers, broccoli, and carrots in 2 tsp. sunflower oil until vegetables are tender, about 6 minutes. Stir in 2 tsp. reduced-sodium soy sauce.* (4)

1/2 c. cooked brown rice (2)

1 c. sliced cucumbers with 1/2 tsp. rice vinegar, salt and pepper to taste (0)

1 c. Bing cherries (1)

**SNACKS** (3 POINTS)

1 c. light apple pie yogurt mixed with 1/4 c. chopped dried apples (3)

1 c. raw mushrooms (0)

**TOTAL DAILY POINTS: 24**

# Day 24 ≡

**BREAKFAST** (6 POINTS)

Sweet Berry Cereal
> *Top 1 c. cooked cream of wheat cereal with 1 tsp. each salt-free butter and packed dark brown sugar; sprinkle with 2 tbsp. dried cranberries and 1 tbsp. wheat germ. Serve with 2 tbsp. half-and-half.* (5)

1 c. blueberries (1)

Coffee or tea (0)

**LUNCH** (4 POINTS)

Shrimp Salad
> *Toss together 1 c. chopped cooked shrimp, 1/3 c. chopped celery, 2 tsp. reduced-calorie mayonnaise, 1 tsp. chopped dill and 1 tsp. lemon juice. Serve over 1 c. mixed greens.* (3)

1 slice (1 oz.) high-fiber whole-wheat bread (1)

1 c. sliced English cucumber (0)

1 c. sugar-free lemonade (0)

**DINNER** (9 POINTS)

Curried Beef Kebabs
> *Combine 4 ounces cubed lean beef, 1 quartered small onion, 1 tsp. sunflower oil, and 1/2 tsp. curry powder. Thread beef and onions on a 12-inch skewer and grill or broil 12 minutes, turning occasionally.* (5.5)

1 c. steamed sugar snap peas topped with 1/2 tsp. salt-free butter (0.5)

1 c. nonfat milk (2)

1 c. baby carrots (1)

**SNACKS** (5 POINTS)

1 1/2 c. sliced fresh strawberries with 1/2 c. fat-free chocolate frozen yogurt (3)

1/2 c. tomato juice (0)

1 c. fat-free milk (2)

**TOTAL DAILY POINTS: 24**

# Day 25 ≣

**BREAKFAST** (6 POINTS)

Maui Muffin
> *Combine 1 c. fresh, cubed pineapple chunks, 1/3 c. low-fat (1%) cottage cheese, and 1 tsp. lemon juice in a blender until smooth. Spread on a toasted oat-bran English muffin.* (4)

1 c. light coconut cream pie yogurt (2)

Coffee or tea (0)

**LUNCH** (5 POINTS)

Mozzarella-Tomato Melt
> *Layer 1/4 c. shredded part-skim mozzarella cheese and 1/2 sliced medium tomato between 2 slices (2 oz.) high-fiber whole-wheat bread spread with 2 tsp. reduced-calorie mayonnaise mixed with 1/2 tsp. chopped basil; broil until bubbly.* (5)

1 c. baby field greens with 1 tsp. balsamic vinegar and salt and pepper to taste (0)

Lemon-lime seltzer (0)

**DINNER** (8 POINTS)

Peppered Steak on Garlic Toast with Cherry Tomato Salsa* (6)

1 c. steamed green beans (0)

1 1/2 c. chopped romaine tossed with 1/2 c. grapefruit sections and 1 tsp. walnut oil (2)

**SNACKS** (3 POINTS)

Hot Mocha
> *In a small saucepan, heat 1 c. fat-free milk, 1 1/2 tsp. unsweetened cocoa powder, and 1 c. coffee; whisk until frothy. Serve with a dusting of cocoa powder.* (2)

2 purple plums (1)

**TOTAL DAILY POINTS: 22**

> *Recipe on page 207.*

# Day 26 ≡

### BREAKFAST (7 POINTS)

Blueberry Belgian Waffle

*Top 1 toasted frozen Belgian waffle with 1 c. blueberries, 3 pecan halves, and 1 tbsp. maple syrup. (5)*

1 c. orange juice (2)

Coffee or tea (0)

### LUNCH (9 POINTS)

Seafood Salad

*Halve 1 tomato lengthwise; squeeze out seeds and drain on paper towels for 10 minutes. Combine 1/2 c. cooked orzo pasta, 1/2 c. imitation crabmeat, 1/4 c. crumbled feta cheese, 10 chopped oil-cured small olives, and 1 tsp. balsamic vinegar. Stuff into tomato halves. (8)*

1 oz. whole-wheat pita, toasted (1)

Lemon-lime seltzer (0)

### DINNER (9 POINTS)

Vegetable Burrito

*Heat 1 tsp. sunflower oil in a medium nonstick skillet. Sauté 1/4 c. cooked black beans with 1/2 c. each chopped tomato, spinach, and mushrooms; add 1/2 c. corn kernels and 1 tsp. fresh chopped cilantro. Remove from heat and combine with 1/4 c. cooked brown rice. Spoon mixture onto heated 6-inch whole-wheat flour tortilla and top with 1/2 c. shredded lettuce and 1/4 c. salsa. (6)*

Raspberries and Cream Shake

*In a blender, combine 1/2 c. fat-free plain yogurt, 1 c. raspberries, 1/4 c. fat-free milk, 2 drops vanilla extract, and 3 ice cubes. Add noncaloric sweetener to taste. (3)*

### SNACKS (3 POINTS)

1/2 c. fat-free sugar-free vanilla pudding made with fat-free milk (1)

1 banana (2)

### TOTAL DAILY POINTS: 28

# Day 27 ≡

**BREAKFAST (5 POINTS)**

$1^1/2$ c. bran-flakes cereal topped with $^1/2$ c. unsweetened canned sliced peaches (3)

1 c. fat-free milk (2)

Coffee or tea (0)

**LUNCH (7 POINTS)**

Potato and Pepper Frittata* (3)

1 c. cantaloupe cubes (1)

Mimosa

*Combine $^1/2$ c. freshly squeezed orange juice with $^1/2$ c. champagne in a 10-oz. wineglass; garnish with 1 fresh strawberry. (3)*

**DINNER (10 POINTS)**

1 c. miso soup (2)

2 c. mixed salad greens with 1 tsp. each rice vinegar and sesame oil (1)

8 pieces maki sushi (4)

$^1/2$ c. green tea ice cream (3)

**SNACKS (4 POINTS)**

1 fat-free apple-cinnamon cereal bar (2)

1 c. fat-free milk (2)

**TOTAL DAILY POINTS: 26**

*Recipe on page 169.*

# Day 28 ≡

## BREAKFAST (5 POINTS)

Fruit and Cream Cereal
> *Stir 1 1/2 tbsp. strawberry spreadable fruit into 1 c. prepared cream of wheat; top with 2 tbsp. half-and-half.* (4)

1 c. sliced strawberries (1)

Coffee or tea (0)

## LUNCH (7 POINTS)

Italian Bread Pizza* (3)

Mixed Salad
> *Toss 1 c. steamed broccoli florets with 1 tsp. each red wine vinegar and sunflower oil. Top with 1 tsp. sunflower seeds. Serve warm or cold.* (1)

3 pickled hot peppers (0)

1 c. light black-cherry yogurt mixed with 1 c. pitted cherries (3)

## DINNER (6.5 POINTS)

Barbecued Chicken
> *Whisk together 2 tsp. ketchup, 1 tsp. each hoisin sauce and cider vinegar, 1/2 tsp. molasses, and 1/2 tsp. reduced-sodium soy sauce; brush onto a 3 oz. skinless, boneless chicken breast. Broil until cooked through, about 5 minutes on each side.* (3)

Dilled Potato Salad
> *Toss together 1 c. chopped cooked new potatoes, 1/2 c. each shredded carrot and chopped scallions, 1/4 c. light plain yogurt, 1 tsp. reduced-calorie mayonnaise, and 1 tsp. chopped dill.* (3.5)

10 cherry tomatoes (0)

Unsweetened iced tea (0)

## SNACKS (6.5 POINTS)

1 c. fat-free milk with 1 tbsp. reduced-calorie chocolate syrup (2.5)

22 roasted salted almonds (4)

## TOTAL DAILY POINTS: 25

*Recipe on page 170.

# 9

## Breakfasts and Brunches

# Lemon-Blueberry Muffins

≡

These delicate crumb-topped, lemon-scented muffins, packed with blueberries, pair well with a cup of tea for a satisfying breakfast or midafternoon snack. If you are using frozen blueberries, toss them into the batter while they are still frozen.

### Makes 12 servings

1 3/4 cups plus 3 tablespoons all-purpose flour
2/3 cup plus 2 tablespoons sugar
2 tablespoons reduced-calorie margarine
1/2 teaspoon ground cinnamon
2 1/4 teaspoons baking powder
1/4 teaspoon baking soda
1/2 teaspoon salt
2 tablespoons cold butter, cut into pieces
2/3 cup low-fat (1%) milk
1/4 cup fat-free egg substitute
1/4 cup unsweetened applesauce
2 teaspoons grated lemon rind
1 teaspoon lemon extract
1 cup fresh or frozen blueberries

1. To prepare the topping, combine the 3 tablespoons flour, 2 tablespoons sugar, the margarine, and the cinnamon in a small bowl; set aside.
2. Preheat the oven to 400° F. Spray a 12-cup muffin tin with nonstick spray or line with foil or paper liners.
3. To prepare the muffins, combine the remaining 1 3/4 cups flour, the remaining 2/3 cup sugar, the baking powder, baking soda, and salt in a large bowl. Add the butter and, with a fork or your fingers, combine the butter with the dry ingredients until the mixture is crumbly.
4. Combine the milk, egg substitute, applesauce, lemon rind, and lemon extract in another bowl. Add the milk mixture to the flour mixture; stir just until blended. Stir in the blueberries.
5. Spoon the batter into the muffin cups, filling each about two-thirds full. Sprinkle the batter with the topping. Bake until the tops of the muffins are golden brown and a toothpick inserted in a muffin comes out clean, about 20 minutes. Cool in the pan on a rack 10 minutes; remove from the pan and cool completely on the rack.

■ **PER SERVING (1 MUFFIN):** 169 calories, 3 g total fat, 1 g saturated fat, 6 mg cholesterol, 265 mg sodium, 32 g total carbohydrates, 1 g dietary fiber, 3 g protein, 75 mg calcium ■ *POINTS PER SERVING: 3*

# Waffles with Goat Cheese, Dried Fruit, and Almonds

eep these ingredients on hand for a speedy, energy-boosting breakfast or snack.

### MAKES 1 SERVING

1 teaspoon goat cheese or light cream cheese (Neufchâtel)
1 frozen multigrain waffle, toasted
1 tablespoon dried cranberries, blueberries, or raisins
1 teaspoon sliced almonds

Spread the cheese on the waffle. Top with the fruit and almonds.

■ **PER SERVING (1 WAFFLE):** 109 calories, 4 g total fat, 1 g saturated fat, 11 mg cholesterol, 192 mg sodium, 16 g total carbohydrates, 1 g dietary fiber, 3 g protein, 50 mg calcium ■ *POINTS: 2*

# Corn and Pepper Pancakes

**P**ancakes are best eaten at once, but this is not always practical when the family wants to eat together. So keep the pancakes warm in a slow oven as you cook them, then eat them as soon as possible. Applesauce or chutney makes a delicious accompaniment to these savory pancakes.

MAKES 4 SERVINGS

3/4 cup all-purpose flour

1/4 cup toasted wheat germ

1 teaspoon sugar

1 teaspoon baking powder

1 teaspoon salt

1/4 teaspoon ground pepper

2 large eggs

1 cup fat-free milk

2 ears fresh corn, kernels removed, or 1 cup frozen corn kernels, thawed

1 small red bell pepper, seeded and finely chopped

1 shallot, minced

1/4 cup chopped fresh parsley

1 1/2 teaspoons canola oil

1. Combine the flour, wheat germ, sugar, baking powder, salt, and ground pepper in a bowl. Combine the eggs, milk, corn, bell pepper, shallot, and parsley in another bowl. Stir the egg mixture into the flour mixture just until blended.

2. Heat 1/2 teaspoon of the oil in a large nonstick skillet or griddle until a drop of water sizzles. Pour the batter by 1/4-cup measures into the skillet. Cook just until bubbles begin to appear at the edges of the pancakes, 2–3 minutes. Flip and cook 2 minutes longer. Repeat with the remaining oil and batter, making a total of 12 pancakes.

■ **PER SERVING (3 PANCAKES):** 239 calories, 6 g total fat, 1 g saturated fat, 107 mg cholesterol, 777 mg sodium, 37 g total carbohydrates, 3 g dietary fiber, 11 g protein, 175 mg calcium ■ *POINTS PER SERVING: 5*

*Tip:* If available, fresh corn on the cob is far superior to frozen corn. Here's an easy way to remove the kernels: After removing the husks and silks from the corn, stand the cob upright on a chopping board. Then, using a sharp knife, cut the kernels down away from the cobs. One ear of corn yields about 1/2 cup of kernels.

# Skillet Apple and Raisin Pancake

T his recipe is traditionally baked in a cast-iron skillet. If you don't have one, just make sure the handle of your skillet is ovenproof, or cover it with heavy-duty foil before putting it in the oven. Be creative using different combinations of fruits. Try a delicious mix of apples and pears, or peaches and plums.

MAKES 6 SERVINGS

1 tablespoon butter
4 Granny Smith apples, peeled, cored, and thinly sliced
$^1/_4$ cup golden raisins
$^1/_4$ cup apple juice
2 tablespoons sugar
$^1/_4$ teaspoon ground cinnamon
1 teaspoon vanilla extract
1 cup low-fat (1%) milk
2 large eggs
2 egg whites
$^1/_4$ teaspoon salt
1 cup all-purpose flour
Confectioners' sugar for dusting

1. Preheat the oven to 425° F.
2. Melt the butter in a large ovenproof skillet, then add the apples, raisins, apple juice, 1 tablespoon of the sugar, and the cinnamon. Cook over medium-high heat, stirring frequently, until the apples are tender and the liquid has evaporated, about 10 minutes. Stir in the vanilla extract. Remove from the heat.
3. Beat together the milk, eggs, egg whites, salt, and the remaining 1 tablespoon sugar in a medium bowl. Gradually whisk in the flour until blended and smooth. Pour the batter over the hot apple mixture. Bake 20 minutes. Reduce the oven temperature to 350° F; bake until puffed and golden, about 15 minutes longer. Sprinkle with the confectioners' sugar. Serve warm or at room temperature.

■ PER SERVING (1/6 PANCAKE): 233 calories, 5 g total fat, 2 g saturated fat, 78 mg cholesterol, 171 mg sodium, 42 g total carbohydrates, 2 g dietary fiber, 7 g protein, 71 mg calcium ■ *POINTS PER SERVING: 5*

*Tip:* For an easy way to core apples, cut the apple in half and use a melon baller to scoop out the core and pits.

# Puffed Egg White Omelet with Peppers and Onions

≡

The trick to making filled omelets taste great is to make sure the vegetables are well cooked. By doing this, the liquid in the vegetables evaporates and the natural sugars are released. When separating the eggs for this omelet, keep five of them in a small bowl and the remaining five, which will be beaten separately, in a large bowl.

MAKES 4 SERVINGS

2 teaspoons olive oil
1 green bell pepper, seeded and thinly sliced
1 red bell pepper, seeded and thinly sliced
1 onion, thinly sliced
1/2 teaspoon salt
10 egg whites, at room temperature
1/2 cup shredded reduced-fat cheddar cheese

1. Heat the oil in a large ovenproof nonstick skillet, then add the green and red bell peppers, the onion, and 1/4 teaspoon of the salt. Cook over medium-high heat, stirring occasionally, until the peppers and onion are very tender, about 8 minutes. Slowly pour in 5 of the egg whites; sprinkle with the cheese. Cook over medium heat, stirring gently, until slightly firm, 3–5 minutes. Remove from the heat.
2. Preheat the broiler.
3. With an electric mixer at high speed, beat the remaining 5 egg whites and the remaining 1/2 teaspoon salt in a large bowl until soft peaks form, 3–4 minutes. Spoon over the pepper mixture to cover completely. Place under the broiler, 7 inches from the heat, until puffed and just golden, about 5 minutes. Cut into wedges. Serve at once.

■ PER SERVING (1/4 OMELET): 122 calories, 4 g total fat, 2 g saturated fat, 8 mg cholesterol, 504 mg sodium, 6 g total carbohydrates, 2 g dietary fiber, 14 g protein, 117 mg calcium ■ *POINTS PER SERVING: 2*

*Tip:* If the handle on your skillet is not ovenproof, cover it with heavy-duty foil.

# Creamed Corn and Cheddar Soufflé

T he variations on this soufflé are endless. If you like, add some chopped Canadian bacon or chopped frozen spinach, thawed and squeezed dry. Serve this with a garden salad for a delicious, satisfying brunch.

MAKES 4 SERVINGS

2 cups low-fat (1%) milk
1 tablespoon butter
1/2 cup cornmeal
1 (14.75-ounce) can creamed corn
1 cup shredded reduced-fat cheddar cheese
4 egg yolks
4 egg whites, at room temperature
1/4 teaspoon cream of tartar

1. Bring the milk and butter to a boil in a large nonstick saucepan over medium-high heat. Slowly add the cornmeal in a thin, steady stream, whisking constantly. Reduce the heat and continue stirring until the mixture is thickened and smooth, about 5 minutes. Remove the pan from the heat and stir in the corn and cheese. Add the egg yolks, one at a time, stirring until blended. Transfer the mixture to a bowl and let cool slightly.
2. Preheat the oven to 375° F. Spray a 2-quart baking dish with nonstick spray.
3. With an electric mixer at high speed, beat the egg whites until foamy; add the cream of tartar and beat until stiff but not grainy. Stir one-fourth of the egg whites into the cornmeal mixture. Fold in the remaining egg whites with a rubber spatula. Scrape the mixture into the baking dish. Bake until puffed and cooked through, about 35 minutes. Serve at once.

■ PER SERVING (1/4 SOUFFLÉ): 380 calories, 15 g total fat, 7 g saturated fat, 241 mg cholesterol, 630 mg sodium, 40 g total carbohydrates, 3 g dietary fiber, 22 g protein, 388 mg calcium ■ *POINTS PER SERVING: 8*

*Tip:* To create more volume in the egg whites, allow them to come to room temperature before you beat them. Make sure to use a large rubber spatula when folding the egg whites into the corn mixture; cut down to the bottom of the bowl, lift and turn the whites over, turning the bowl as you go.

# Potato and Pepper Frittata

A frittata is the ultimate easy-on-the-cook brunch dish. Here, I use a classic mixture of potatoes, peppers, and cheddar cheese, but you could substitute other vegetables, such as zucchini, chopped broccoli, or tomatoes, and other cheeses, such as feta or Monterey Jack.

MAKES 4 SERVINGS

1 tablespoon canola oil
2 cups (from a 32-ounce bag) frozen hash brown potatoes
1 bunch scallions, thinly sliced
1 red bell pepper, seeded and chopped
3/4 teaspoon salt
1/4 cup chopped flat-leaf parsley
2 cups fat-free egg substitute, thawed
1/2 cup shredded reduced-fat cheddar cheese
1 tablespoon shredded Parmesan cheese
1/2 teaspoon coarsely ground black pepper

1. Heat the oil in a medium nonstick skillet, then add the hash browns, scallions, bell pepper, and salt. Cook over medium heat, stirring frequently, until the vegetables are tender and golden, 8–10 minutes.
2. Meanwhile, spray a large nonstick skillet with nonstick spray and set over medium heat. Add the egg substitute and cook until set, 7–8 minutes, lifting the edges frequently with a spatula to let the uncooked egg flow underneath.
3. Spoon the potato mixture over the frittata, then sprinkle with the cheddar cheese, Parmesan cheese, and pepper. Cover the skillet and cook until the cheese melts, about 3 minutes.

■ **PER SERVING (1/4 FRITTATA):** 190 calories, 4 g total fat, 1 g saturated fat, 1 mg cholesterol, 653 mg sodium, 26 g total carbohydrates, 4 g dietary fiber, 13 g protein, 98 mg calcium ■ *POINTS PER SERVING: 3*

*Tip:* For a browned cheese topping, pop the frittata under a hot broiler for 2–3 minutes. If the handle on your skillet is not flameproof, cover it with heavy-duty foil.

# 10

## Light Bites and Appetizers

## Italian Bread Pizzas

≡

This easy snack will zap any late-day hunger pangs. You can substitute arugula if fresh basil isn't available.

MAKES 6 SERVINGS

1 (8-ounce) loaf Italian bread
1 large tomato, cut into thin slices
1 garlic clove, minced
1/2 teaspoon salt
1/2 cup shredded part-skim mozzarella cheese
1/4 cup chopped fresh basil
2 teaspoons dried oregano

1. Preheat the broiler.
2. Slice the bread lengthwise, then cut each in thirds crosswise to make 6 pieces. Arrange the tomato on the bread pieces and sprinkle with the garlic and salt. Top with the mozzarella, basil, and oregano. Place the pizzas on the broiler rack.
3. Broil 6 inches from the heat until the cheese is melted and bubbly, about 3 minutes.

■ PER SERVING (1 SLICE): 137 calories, 3 g total fat, 1 g saturated fat, 5 mg cholesterol, 467 mg sodium, 21 g total carbohydrates, 2 g dietary fiber, 6 g protein, 108 mg calcium ■ POINTS PER SERVING: 3

# Portobello and Onion Toasts

≡

arge and meaty, portobello mushrooms are actually full-grown cremini mushrooms. They are delicious in sandwiches and salads. Fontina is a semisoft, creamy cow's milk cheese that melts easily and has a mild, nutty flavor. For best flavor, choose Italian fontina cheese if you can get it. Alternatively, substitute shredded reduced-fat cheddar, or mozzarella cheese.

### MAKES 4 SERVINGS

2 teaspoons olive oil

3/4 pound fresh portobello mushrooms, stems removed and sliced

1 onion, thinly sliced

1 garlic clove, chopped

1/4 teaspoon salt

1/4 cup dry vermouth

4 (1/2-inch thick) slices Italian bread, toasted

1/4 cup shredded fontina cheese

1. Heat the oil in a large nonstick skillet, then add the mushrooms, onion, garlic, and salt. Cook over medium-high heat, stirring occasionally, until the mushrooms and onion are very tender, about 8 minutes. Stir in the vermouth and cook over medium heat, stirring occasionally, until the mushrooms and onions are golden brown and any liquid has evaporated, about 5 minutes.

2. Preheat the broiler.

3. Spoon the mushroom mixture onto the toasted bread. Sprinkle with the cheese. Broil, 4 inches from the heat, until the cheese is melted and bubbly, about 4 minutes. Serve at once.

■ PER SERVING (1 TOAST): 141 calories, 5 g total fat, 2 g saturated fat, 6 mg cholesterol, 310 mg sodium, 18 g total carbohydrates, 2 g dietary fiber, 5 g protein, 76 mg calcium ■ *POINTS PER SERVING: 3*

≡

# Vegetarian Nachos

When you're ready for a quiet night at home watching a favorite movie, here's a popular snack the whole family will appreciate. Substitute black beans for the pinto beans, if you prefer. For a spicier version, add some minced jalapeños and use hot salsa instead of mild.

MAKES 6 SERVINGS

1 (15-ounce) can pinto beans, rinsed and drained
1 (8-ounce) can corn kernels, drained
2 tablespoons (from a 4-ounce can) chopped green chilis
1 tablespoon chili powder
1/2 teaspoon ground cumin
1/2 cup shredded reduced-fat sharp cheddar cheese
2 cups low-fat baked tortilla chips
2 cups shredded romaine lettuce
1 tomato, chopped
1/4 cup light sour cream
1/4 cup mild salsa
2 tablespoons chopped pitted ripe olives
2 tablespoons chopped fresh cilantro (optional)

1. Combine the beans, corn, chilis, chili powder, and cumin in a medium nonstick saucepan. Cook over medium heat, stirring frequently, until hot. Stir in the cheese until melted.

2. Arrange the tortilla chips on a large plate. Spoon the bean mixture over the chips, then top with the lettuce, tomato, sour cream, salsa, olives, and cilantro (if using). Serve at once.

■ **PER SERVING (1/6 OF THE NACHOS):** 174 calories, 4 g total fat, 2 g saturated fat, 8 mg cholesterol, 394 mg sodium, 28 g total carbohydrates, 6 g dietary fiber, 9 g protein, 125 mg calcium ■ *POINTS PER SERVING: 3*

# Corn Dogs

Y ou won't have to wait for the carnival to come to town to enjoy these tasty corn dogs, nor will you want to. Our lean version looks and tastes just like the original. Just for fun, serve them on popsicle sticks.

MAKES 8 SERVINGS

1/4 cup reduced-fat baking mix
1/4 cup low-fat (1%) milk
6 tablespoons cornflake crumbs
1/2 (14-ounce) package reduced-fat beef hot dogs (4 hot dogs)

1. Preheat the oven to 425° F. Spray a baking sheet with nonstick spray.
2. Combine the baking mix and milk in a pie plate until blended. Place the cornflake crumbs on a sheet of wax paper. Dip the hot dogs into the baking mix mixture, then roll in the crumbs. Place the hot dogs on the baking sheet. Spray lightly with nonstick spray. Bake until the hot dogs are heated through and the crust is golden brown, about 15 minutes. Cut in half and serve at once.

■ PER SERVING (1/2 CORN DOG): 87 calories, 5 g total fat, 2 g saturated fat, 17 mg cholesterol, 340 mg sodium, 5 g total carbohydrates, 0 g dietary fiber, 5 g protein, 18 mg calcium ■ POINTS PER SERVING: 2

# Tortilla Pinwheels

Like a chef's salad rolled up in a tortilla, these pinwheels are a tasty treat. If you like, substitute sliced turkey breast for the ham. You can use any leafy greens you have on hand in place of the spinach.

MAKES 4 SERVINGS

1 cup torn fresh spinach
1/2 tomato, chopped
1/4 small onion, thinly sliced
1 1/2 teaspoons cider vinegar
2 (6-inch) fat-free flour tortillas, warmed
2 ounces light cream cheese (Neufchâtel)
2 tablespoons sliced pimiento-stuffed green olives
3 ounces sliced fat-free turkey ham

1. Combine the spinach, tomato, onion, and vinegar in a medium bowl.
2. Heat each tortilla in a dry skillet until softened and warm. Stack the tortillas between sheets of paper towels and cover with plastic wrap to prevent from drying out; set aside.
3. Spread the cream cheese onto the tortillas. Top with the olives, then the spinach mixture and ham. Roll the tortillas and cut each one into 6 pieces, making a total of 12 pinwheels. Serve at once or refrigerate, covered, until ready to serve.

■ **PER SERVING (3 PINWHEELS):** 109 calories, 5 g total fat, 3 g saturated fat, 23 mg cholesterol, 459 mg sodium, 8 g total carbohydrates, 1 g dietary fiber, 7 g protein, 46 mg calcium ■ *POINTS PER SERVING: 2*

# White Bean Dip

≡

This luscious dip is ideal for everyday snacking with plenty of crunchy, no-point veggies such as celery and carrot sticks, bell pepper strips, steamed broccoli or cauliflower florets, and Belgian endive leaves. It also makes a delicious sandwich spread for whole-wheat pita breads. The dip keeps in the refrigerator for up to 3 days.

### MAKES 4 SERVINGS

1 (15$^1$/2-ounce) can white beans, rinsed and drained
2 garlic cloves, chopped
1 tablespoon extravirgin olive oil
$^3$/4 teaspoon ground cumin
$^1$/2 teaspoon salt
$^1$/4 teaspoon ground pepper

Process the beans, garlic, oil, cumin, salt, and pepper in a food processor until smooth. Transfer the mixture to a medium bowl and refrigerate, covered, until ready to serve.

■ **PER SERVING (1/4 CUP):** 138 calories, 4 g total fat, 1 g saturated fat, 0 mg cholesterol, 472 mg sodium, 20 g total carbohydrates, 5 g dietary fiber, 7 g protein, 74 mg calcium ■ *POINTS PER SERVING: 2*

≡

# Avocado Boats with Salsa

This is a fiber- and vitamin-filled treat for avocado lovers. When they're in season (from November through February), choose Haas avocados from Mexico, with their smooth and creamy, full-flavored flesh. Avocados are rich in fiber, potassium, folic acid and other B vitamins, and vitamin E. Their "good" fats are recommended as part of a heart-healthy diet.

MAKES 8 SERVINGS

1 small tomato, diced
2 tablespoons minced red onion
1 tablespoon chopped fresh cilantro
1 tablespoon red wine vinegar
1/8 teaspoon salt
2 ripe avocados, unpeeled, pitted, and cut in quarters lengthwise
4 teaspoons nonfat sour cream
Fresh cilantro sprigs (optional)

Combine the tomato, onion, cilantro, vinegar, and salt in a small bowl. Spoon the tomato mixture onto the avocado quarters. Top each quarter with the sour cream and cilantro sprigs (if using). Serve at once.

■ PER SERVING (1 FILLED AVOCADO QUARTER): 75 calories, 6 g total fat, 1 g saturated fat, 0 mg cholesterol, 43 mg sodium, 4 g total carbohydrates, 3 g dietary fiber, 1 g protein, 12 mg calcium ■ *POINTS PER SERVING: 1*

*Tip:* An avocado that feels soft when lightly pressed is ripe and ready to eat. If they are not ripe in the store, ripen them for a few days on a counter (speed up the ripening by putting them in a paper bag). To remove the pit, cut the avocado in half lengthwise and twist the two halves apart. With the blade of a large chef's knife, make a quick downward stroke into the pit and twist. The pit will attach itself to the knife and come out.

# Crab Cakes

≡

These delicate cakes also are a delicious way to start a fancy company dinner. Or double the recipe and form them into smallish cakes for bite-sized hors d'oeuvres your guests will love.

MAKES 4 SERVINGS

1 red bell pepper, seeded and coarsely chopped
4 scallions, coarsely chopped
1 celery rib, coarsely chopped
2 large eggs
2 egg whites
2 tablespoons reduced-fat mayonnaise
1 tablespoon Worcestershire sauce
$1/2$ teaspoon crushed red pepper
6 ounces French bread, made into crumbs (3 cups)
$1/2$ pound cooked lump crabmeat, picked over and flaked
2 teaspoons canola oil
4 cups mixed leafy greens, such as mesclun
4 lemon wedges

1. Pulse the bell pepper, scallions, celery, eggs, egg whites, mayonnaise, Worcestershire sauce, and crushed red pepper in a food processor until finely chopped. Transfer to a medium bowl.
2. Stir in the bread crumbs and crabmeat. Cover and refrigerate until the bread absorbs the liquid, at least 10 minutes or up to overnight.
3. Shape the mixture into 12 patties. Heat 1 teaspoon of the oil in a large nonstick skillet, then add 6 patties and cook until golden and heated through, 3–4 minutes on each side. Repeat with the remaining oil and patties.
4. Serve the crab cakes on the mixed greens with the lemon wedges.

■ **PER SERVING (3 CRAB CAKES AND 1 CUP MESCLUN):** 291 calories, 10 g total fat, 2 g saturated fat, 165 mg cholesterol, 596 mg sodium, 28 g total carbohydrates, 4 g dietary fiber, 22 g protein, 167 mg calcium ■ *POINTS PER SERVING: 6*

# California Sushi Rolls

Sushi is surprisingly easy to make at home. Most of the ingredients, including sushi rice (a short-grain rice), rice vinegar, wasabi powder (green horseradish powder), and nori (paper-thin sheets of dried seaweed, rich in protein, calcium, and iron) can be found in Asian markets. Surimi, sometimes called imitation crabmeat, is a common filling used in California rolls. It's actually pressed pollock or whiting and has a delicate, slightly sweet flavor. Surimi is available in the seafood section of your supermarket. You will need a bamboo rolling mat to roll the sushi. These mats are easily found in kitchen stores or Asian markets. Serve the rolls with pickled ginger if you like.

MAKES 6 SERVINGS

$2^1/_4$ cups water

2 cups sushi rice, rinsed

$^1/_2$ cup seasoned rice vinegar

1 tablespoon toasted sesame seeds

3 tablespoons warm water

2 tablespoons reduced-sodium soy sauce

2 teaspoons wasabi powder

1 teaspoon Asian (dark) sesame oil

1 teaspoon grated peeled fresh ginger

4 (7 × 8-inch) nori sheets

$^1/_2$ cucumber, peeled and cut into thin strips

$^1/_2$ avocado, peeled, pitted and cut into thin strips

4 ounces surimi, cut into thin strips

1. Bring the water and rice to a boil in a medium saucepan. Reduce the heat and simmer, covered, until the rice is tender and the liquid is absorbed, about 20 minutes. Transfer the rice to a large bowl. Stir in the vinegar and sesame seeds. Let stand until cool enough to handle.

2. Meanwhile, to prepare the wasabi dipping sauce, whisk together the water, soy sauce, wasabi powder, sesame oil, and ginger until blended. Set aside.

3. Place a sheet of nori lengthwise, shiny side down, onto the rolling mat. Dampen your hands with water and spread 1 cup of the rice mixture onto the nori, leaving a half-inch border across the top. Make a $^1/_4$-inch-deep indentation crosswise along the cen-

ter of the rice for the filling. Place $^1/_4$ each of the cucumber, avocado, and surimi into the groove of the rice.

4. Hold the filling in place with your fingers as you curl the mat forward with your thumbs until the two ends of the nori overlap, forming a cylinder. Applying gentle but even pressure to the rolling mat, remove the roll from the mat. Cut into six pieces with a very sharp knife, moistening the knife with water, between each cut. Repeat with the remaining nori, rice, cucumber, avocado, and surimi. Serve the rolls with the dipping sauce.

■ **PER SERVING (4 ROLLS):** 314 calories, 4 g total fat, 1 g saturated fat, 6 mg cholesterol, 381 mg sodium, 59 g total carbohydrates, 3 g dietary fiber, 9 g protein, 38 mg calcium ■ *POINTS PER SERVING: 6*

# 11
## Lunches

# Cock-a-Leekie

T he name of this soothing Scottish soup literally translates as "chicken and leeks." Prunes are traditionally added for a touch of sweetness, but the sweetest thing of all is that this homemade chicken soup can be on the table in 20 minutes. Serve this soup with four slices of oat-bran bread, toasted and cut into triangles (it adds an extra 2 points to each serving).

MAKES 4 SERVINGS

1 teaspoon canola oil
1 1/4 pounds leeks, cleaned and thinly sliced
6 cups low-sodium chicken broth
2/3 cup quick-cooking barley
2 parsnips, finely chopped
1/2 teaspoon ground pepper
3/4 pound skinless boneless chicken breasts, cut into 1-inch pieces
1/2 pound white mushrooms, sliced
6 pitted prunes, chopped
1 teaspoon dried thyme
2 tablespoons port or sherry

1. Heat the oil in a nonstick Dutch oven, then add the leeks. Cook over medium heat, stirring occasionally, until softened, 7–8 minutes. Add the broth, barley, parsnips, and pepper; bring to a boil. Reduce the heat and simmer, covered, about 8 minutes.

2. Add the chicken, mushrooms, prunes, and thyme; return to a boil. Reduce the heat and simmer, covered, until the chicken is just cooked through, 3–4 minutes. Stir in the port or sherry.

■ **PER SERVING (A GENEROUS 2 CUPS):** 387 calories, 6 g total fat, 1 g saturated fat, 46 mg cholesterol, 149 mg sodium, 55 g total carbohydrates, 11 g dietary fiber, 29 g protein, 115 mg calcium ■ *POINTS PER SERVING: 7*

*Tip:* Leeks often contain sand in between their layers. Here's how to clean them: Trim away most of the dark green tops and the roots, leaving the root end intact to hold the layers together. Slice the leek lengthwise to within a half inch of the root end. Hold the leek by the root end, fan open the layers, and rinse thoroughly under cold running water.

# Italian Bread Soup with Escarole

≡

Pancetta (pan-*cheh*-tuh), a flavorful Italian bacon in a sausagelike shape, is found in specialty food stores. Tightly wrapped, it keeps in the refrigerator for up to 3 weeks and in the freezer for up to 6 months.

## MAKES 4 SERVINGS

2 tablespoons chopped pancetta
1 onion, chopped
3 garlic cloves, minced
4 cups low-sodium vegetable or chicken broth
1 (14-ounce) can Italian cherry tomatoes
1 bunch escarole, cleaned and chopped (about 5 cups)
1 1/2 tablespoons chopped fresh oregano or 1 1/2 teaspoons dried
1/2 teaspoon ground pepper
2 (15-ounce) cans cannellini (white kidney) beans, rinsed and drained
4 ounces Italian bread, cut into 8 slices
1/3 cup shredded Parmesan cheese

1. Spray a nonstick Dutch oven with nonstick spray and set over medium heat. Add the pancetta and cook until browned, 2–3 minutes; transfer to a plate.
2. Add the onion and garlic to the same Dutch oven. Cook, stirring frequently, until golden, 7–10 minutes. Add the broth, tomatoes, escarole, oregano, and pepper; bring to a boil, stirring occasionally. Reduce the heat and simmer, covered, until the escarole is softened, about 5 minutes. Stir in the beans and cook until hot, 2–3 minutes.
3. Preheat the broiler. Transfer the soup to a large ovenproof casserole dish. Arrange the bread slices on top of the soup; sprinkle with the cheese. Broil until the cheese and bread are lightly browned, 1–2 minutes. Sprinkle with the pancetta just before serving.

■ **PER SERVING (GENEROUS 2 CUPS):** 385 calories, 6 g total fat, 2 g saturated fat, 7 mg cholesterol, 910 mg sodium, 62 g total carbohydrates, 16 g dietary fiber, 23 g protein, 275 mg calcium ■ *POINTS PER SERVING: 7*

# Chili Bean and Cheese Burritos

L ively cilantro and vinegar add sparkle to the tomato-olive topping in these quick, healthy burritos—a terrific way to feed a hungry family of four.

MAKES 4 SERVINGS

1 tomato, chopped
1/4 cup pitted ripe olives, chopped
3 tablespoons chopped fresh cilantro
2 tablespoons red wine vinegar
1/4 teaspoon salt
1 (16-ounce) can fat-free refried beans
3 tablespoons mild, medium, or hot salsa
2 tablespoons (from a 4-ounce can) chopped mild green chilis
1/2 cup shredded Monterey Jack cheese
4 (8-inch) fat-free flour tortillas, warmed
1/4 cup light sour cream

1. Combine the tomato, olives, cilantro, vinegar, and salt in a medium bowl; set aside.
2. Place the beans, salsa, and chilis in a medium nonstick saucepan. Cook over medium heat, stirring occasionally, until heated through, 3–4 minutes. Remove from the heat and stir in the cheese.
3. Spread each warmed tortilla with the bean mixture then top with the tomato mixture and the sour cream. Roll and cut each diagonally in half. If not serving right away, cover with damp paper towels and plastic wrap for up to 15 minutes.

■ **PER SERVING (1 BURRITO):** 300 calories, 7 g total fat, 4 g saturated fat, 18 mg cholesterol, 1,003 mg sodium, 47 g total carbohydrates, 8 g dietary fiber, 14 g protein, 228 mg calcium ■ *POINTS PER SERVING: 6*

*Tip:* To heat the tortillas, put them between layers of damp paper towels and microwave on high (four tortillas should take 35–40 seconds). Keep them covered until ready to use so they won't dry out. To transform the recipe into a delicious appetizer, cut the tortillas into wedges and bake them in a 425° F. oven until crisp, about 8 minutes. Spread the wedges with the bean mixture, then the tomato mixture. Top with a little light sour cream and garnish with cilantro sprigs.

# Southwestern Ham, Cheese, and Potato Casserole

≡

**L**eaving the skins on the potatoes adds a touch of extra fiber to this recipe, while a generous amount of red and green bell peppers contributes a nice vitamin boost. A simple green salad will complete the lunch.

Makes 4 servings

1 teaspoon olive oil
1 red bell pepper, seeded and chopped
1 green bell pepper, seeded and chopped
1 bunch scallions, thinly sliced
1 cup cherry tomatoes, quartered
1/4 pound sliced cooked ham, cut into strips
2 teaspoons chili powder
2 teaspoons ground cumin
1/2 teaspoon ground pepper
2 baking potatoes, scrubbed and thinly sliced
1/2 cup shredded reduced-fat cheddar cheese

1. Preheat the oven to 350° F. Spray an 8-inch-square baking dish with nonstick spray.
2. Heat the oil in a large nonstick skillet, then add the red and green bell peppers and the scallions. Cook over medium-high heat, stirring occasionally, until softened, about 5 minutes. Add the tomatoes, ham, chili powder, cumin, and ground pepper; cook until heated through, about 2 minutes.
3. Spread half of the potatoes in the baking dish, top with half of the bell pepper mixture. Repeat layering once more. Cover with foil and bake until the potatoes are tender, about 45 minutes. Uncover, sprinkle with the cheese, and bake until the cheese is lightly browned, about 10 minutes longer.

■ **PER SERVING (1/4 CASSEROLE):** 231 calories, 7 g total fat, 3 g saturated fat, 24 mg cholesterol, 531 mg sodium, 30 g total carbohydrates, 5 g dietary fiber, 14 g protein, 156 mg calcium ■ *POINTS PER SERVING: 4*

# Roasted Vegetable Pizza

A carbohydrate-packed crust and copious juicy vegetables make this a high-energy, high-fiber lunch. Experiment with whatever veggies strike your fancy: try sliced mushrooms, cubed eggplant, even shredded cabbage and carrots. The spicy, melted, pepper-jack cheese ties it all together deliciously.

MAKES 4 SERVINGS

2 zucchini, cut into 1/2-inch slices
1 yellow bell pepper, seeded and cut into 16 pieces
1 green bell pepper, seeded and cut into 16 pieces
1 small red onion, peeled and cut into 8 wedges
2 plum tomatoes, sliced
1 (10-ounce) package thin pizza crust
1 cup shredded reduced-fat pepper-jack cheese

1. Preheat the oven to 450° F. Spray a large nonstick roasting pan with nonstick spray. Place the zucchini, yellow and green bell peppers, red onion, and tomatoes in the roasting pan in a single layer; spray lightly with nonstick spray. Roast until softened and lightly browned, about 25 minutes.

2. Place the pizza crust on a baking sheet. Spread the roasted vegetables on the crust. Sprinkle with the cheese and bake until hot and the cheese is lightly browned, 7–8 minutes.

■ PER SERVING (1/4 PIZZA): 314 calories, 9 g total fat, 4 g saturated fat, 15 mg cholesterol, 484 mg sodium, 43 g total carbohydrates, 4 g dietary fiber, 15 g protein, 238 mg calcium ■ *POINTS PER SERVING: 6*

*Tip:* It's important to roast vegetables in a single layer in the roasting pan. This will prevent the vegetables from steaming and encourage them to brown and caramelize. If necessary, use 2 pans.

# Roast Beef Sandwich with Roasted Garlic Aïoli

 ïoli, a strong garlic mayonnaise from Provence in the south of France, is made here with very little fat, but with lots of mellow flavor from roasted garlic. Feel free to use it as a spread for other hearty sandwiches, such as roast pork or turkey.

MAKES 4 SERVINGS

1 whole garlic bulb
2 tablespoons plain nonfat yogurt
2 tablespoons reduced-fat mayonnaise
2 teaspoons extravirgin olive oil
1/4 teaspoon ground pepper
1 (8-ounce) French baguette, split in half lengthwise
1/2 pound thinly sliced lean roast beef or turkey
1 cup arugula leaves
2 tomatoes, sliced

1. To make the roasted garlic aïoli, preheat the oven to 450° F. Wrap the garlic bulb in foil and roast until fragrant and softened, 25–30 minutes. Let cool 15 minutes. Cut the top from the garlic and squeeze the garlic pulp into a small bowl. Stir in the yogurt, mayonnaise, oil, and pepper.
2. Spread the aïoli on both sides of the baguette. Layer the roast beef, arugula, and tomatoes on one side of the baguette. Top with the remaining baguette half and cut into 4 pieces.

   ■ PER SERVING (1/4 SANDWICH): 330 calories, 10 g total fat, 2 g saturated fat, 50 mg cholesterol, 437 mg sodium, 35 g total carbohydrates, 3 g dietary fiber, 25 g protein, 89 mg calcium ■ POINTS PER SERVING: 7

   *Tip:* Chewing fresh parsley is helpful for eliminating garlic odors from the breath. For a milder garlic taste, substitute 4 cloves of elephant garlic—if you can find it—for the regular garlic.

# Roasted Red Pepper
# and Goat Cheese Sandwich

≡

F or this simple snack, roasted red peppers from a jar or frozen package make a quick
alternative to roasting your own. Flavorful goat cheese, sweet yet sharp red onion, and
pungent basil complement the peppers and crusty rolls.

2 ounces reduced-fat goat cheese
4 crusty rolls, split
1 (12-ounce) jar roasted red peppers, drained
1/2 red onion, thinly sliced
1/2 cup chopped fresh basil

Spread the goat cheese on the bottom half of each roll. Top with the red peppers,
onion, and basil. Replace the tops and serve at once.

■ **PER SERVING (1 SANDWICH):** 208 calories, 5 g total fat, 2 g saturated fat, 13
mg cholesterol, 497 mg sodium, 33 g total carbohydrates, 3 g dietary fiber, 8 g protein, 134 mg calcium ■ *POINTS PER SERVING: 4*

*T i p :* When they're in season, look for sweet Vidalia onions to use instead of
the red onion.

≡

# Lentil and Beet Salad
# with Goat Cheese

≡

**L**ean legumes, such as lentils and beans, are carbohydrate-packed, energy-boosting foods. You can make this salad with any variety of them. If you prefer, substitute 3 cups of drained canned chickpeas or kidney beans for the lentils and omit step 1.

## MAKES 4 SERVINGS

1 cup lentils, picked over, rinsed, and drained

1/2 onion, chopped

4 cups water

3 tablespoons balsamic vinegar

1 tablespoon Dijon mustard

2 teaspoons extravirgin olive oil

1/2 teaspoon salt

1 (15-ounce) can small whole beets, drained and quartered

1 yellow bell pepper, seeded and finely chopped

1/4 cup chopped fresh mint

2 cups torn salad greens

4 ounces reduced-fat goat cheese, crumbled

1. Bring the lentils, onion, and water to a boil. Reduce the heat and simmer, covered, until tender, about 20 minutes. Drain the lentils and set aside.

2. Meanwhile, whisk together the vinegar, mustard, oil, and salt in a large bowl. Add the lentils, beets, yellow pepper, and mint. Arrange the salad greens on a large platter. Spoon the lentil mixture on top. Sprinkle with the goat cheese.

■ **PER SERVING (1 1/2 CUPS):** 295 calories, 9 g total fat, 5 g saturated fat, 25 mg cholesterol, 560 mg sodium, 38 g total carbohydrates, 13 g dietary fiber, 18 g protein, 205 mg calcium ■ *POINTS PER SERVING: 6*

≡

# Shrimp, Fennel, and Grapes in Cantaloupe Halves

≡

**H**ere's an elegant main-dish take on a Waldorf salad, using a delicious mix of succulent shrimp, crunchy fennel, and sweet grapes in a fresh lime dressing. To save time, buy the shrimp precooked at the fish market the day you plan to serve this and omit step 1.

### MAKES 4 SERVINGS

3/4 pound medium shrimp, peeled and deveined
1/2 fennel bulb, trimmed and very thinly sliced, or 1 cup sliced celery
1 cup seedless grapes, halved
2 tablespoons reduced-fat mayonnaise
2 tablespoons chopped fennel leaves
1 tablespoon fresh lime or lemon juice
2 cantaloupes, halved and seeded
2 tablespoons chopped toasted walnuts

1. Bring a pot of water to a boil; add the shrimp and simmer until just opaque in the center, 3–4 minutes. Drain in a colander and rinse under cold water to stop the cooking. Dry the shrimp on paper towels.

2. Combine the shrimp, fennel, grapes, mayonnaise, fennel leaves, and lime juice in a medium bowl. Spoon into the cantaloupe halves, sprinkle with the walnuts, and serve at once.

■ **PER SERVING (1 CANTALOUPE HALF AND 3/4 CUP FILLING):** 289 calories, 7 g total fat, 1 g saturated fat, 82 mg cholesterol, 208 mg sodium, 49 g total carbohydrates, 5 g dietary fiber, 14 g protein, 90 mg calcium ■ *POINTS PER SERVING: 6*

*Tip:* Chopped fennel leaves add flavor to this dish. If you're using celery in place of the fennel, consider adding chopped fresh mint as a substitute for the fennel leaves. To toast the walnuts, place them in a small dry skillet over medium-low heat. Cook, shaking the pan and stirring constantly, until lightly browned and fragrant, 3–4 minutes. Watch them carefully when toasting; walnuts can burn quickly. Transfer the nuts to a plate to cool.

# Wheat Berries with
# Smoked Turkey and Fruit

≡

**W**heat berries are whole, unprocessed wheat kernels that add wonderful crunch and flavor to any salad. You can find them in health food stores and specialty markets. High in protein, they will keep for up to one year in an airtight container stored in a cool, dark and dry space.

MAKES 4 SERVINGS

2 1/4 cups water
1 cup wheat berries, rinsed
1/2 pound smoked turkey in one piece, cubed
2 nectarines, pitted and cubed
1 Granny Smith apple, cored and cubed
1/2 red onion, chopped
1/4 cup orange juice
3 tablespoons cider vinegar
1 tablespoon Dijon mustard
1 tablespoon honey
1/2 (10-ounce) bag fresh baby spinach, cleaned and coarsely chopped

1. Bring the water to a boil in a medium saucepan. Stir in the wheat berries; reduce the heat and simmer, covered, until the berries are tender and the water is absorbed, 1 1/2–2 hours. Fluff the wheat berries with a fork, then let stand 5 minutes.
2. Combine the wheat berries with the turkey, nectarines, apple, and onion in a large bowl. Whisk together the orange juice, vinegar, mustard, and honey in a small bowl. Stir the juice mixture into the wheat berry mixture until blended.
3. Arrange the spinach on a platter. Spoon the wheat berries mixture on top. Serve at once.

■ **PER SERVING (2 CUPS):** 285 calories, 3 g total fat, 1 g saturated fat, 23 mg cholesterol, 765 mg sodium, 54 g total carbohydrates, 9 g dietary fiber, 16 g protein, 66 mg calcium ■ *POINTS PER SERVING: 5*

*Tip:* If you're pressed for time, substitute bulgur wheat (it cooks in about 25 minutes) for the whole wheat berries.

# Pasta Salad Tonnato

This main-dish pasta salad, made with tuna, olives, and capers, is ideal for a summer luncheon, a quick supper, or an easy picnic. It all comes together in a snap with just a few simple staples from your kitchen pantry. Substitute canned salmon for the tuna, if you like.

MAKES 6 SERVINGS

8 ounces penne pasta
1 (12-ounce) can water-packed chunk light tuna, drained
3 celery ribs, finely chopped
1/2 red onion, thinly sliced
10 kalamata olives, pitted and chopped
2 tablespoons capers, drained and chopped
2 teaspoons grated lemon rind
1/3 cup reduced-calorie mayonnaise
2 tablespoons Dijon mustard
1 tablespoon fresh lemon juice
Pinch of cayenne

1. Cook the penne according to the package directions; drain. Rinse under cold running water. Transfer the penne to a large bowl. Add the tuna, celery, onion, olives, capers, and lemon rind.
2. Whisk together the mayonnaise, mustard, lemon juice, and cayenne until blended. Stir the mayonnaise mixture with the pasta mixture until blended.

■ **PER SERVING (1½ CUPS):** 268 calories, 7 g total fat, 1 g saturated fat, 20 mg cholesterol, 490 mg sodium, 33 g total carbohydrates, 2 g dietary fiber, 19 g protein, 35 mg calcium ■ *POINTS PER SERVING: 6*

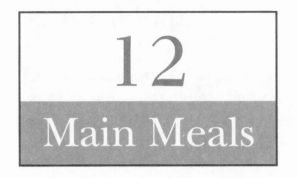

## 12

## Main Meals

# Roast Chicken with Chestnut, Kale, and Dried Cherry Stuffing

≡

**R**oast chestnuts, kale, and dried cherries make a robust stuffing for this classic Sunday roast. The skin is left on the chicken while it roasts, sealing in flavor and moisture. Then, just before carving, the skin is removed. The colorful stuffing is cooked in a separate pan so that it doesn't absorb any fat from the chicken.

### MAKES 6 SERVINGS

1 (3$^1$/$_2$-pound) roasting chicken

$^1$/$_2$ teaspoon salt

1 lemon, quartered

3 large garlic cloves, halved

4 sprigs fresh rosemary or 1 teaspoon dried

2 teaspoons butter

1 red onion, chopped

$^3$/$_4$ cup low-sodium chicken broth

3 cups herb-seasoned stuffing mix

$^1$/$_2$ pound fresh chestnuts, roasted and chopped

$^1$/$_2$ (10-ounce) package frozen chopped kale, thawed and drained

$^1$/$_2$ cup chopped dried cherries or cranberries

2 tablespoons cognac
Fresh rosemary sprigs (optional)

1. Preheat the oven to 400° F. Spray the rack of a roasting pan with nonstick spray and place the rack in the pan. Spray an 8-inch-square baking dish with nonstick spray.
2. Lightly spray the outside of the chicken with nonstick spray and sprinkle with the salt. Place the lemon, garlic, and rosemary inside the cavity of the chicken. Tuck the wings under, then place the chicken, breast side up, on the rack in the roasting pan.
3. Roast the chicken 25 minutes. Reduce the oven temperature to 350° F and roast until the skin is lightly browned and an instant-read thermometer, inserted in the thigh, registers 180° F., about 50 minutes longer.
4. Meanwhile, melt the butter in a large nonstick saucepan, then add the onion. Cook over medium heat, stirring frequently, until softened, 3–5 minutes. Add the broth, stuffing mix, chestnuts, kale, cherries, and cognac; cook, stirring frequently, until hot, 2–3 minutes. Spoon into the baking dish. Cover with foil and bake alongside the chicken 20 minutes; uncover and bake until heated through and the top is lightly browned, about 10 minutes longer.
5. Let the chicken stand 10 minutes. Remove and discard the lemon, garlic, and rosemary. Remove and discard the skin, then carve. Serve with the stuffing. Garnish with the rosemary (if using).

■ **PER SERVING (1/6 CHICKEN AND SCANT 1 CUP STUFFING):** 410 calories, 9 g total fat, 3 g saturated fat, 80 mg cholesterol, 680 mg sodium, 47 g total carbohydrates, 5 g dietary fiber, 33 g protein, 102 mg calcium ■ *POINTS PER SERVING: 8*

*Tip:* To roast chestnuts, preheat the oven to 400° F. With a sharp knife, cut a large X in each chestnut to allow the steam to escape. Spread on a baking sheet and roast until the slits open, about 20 minutes. Remove from the oven and cover with a damp towel for 5 minutes to steam the chestnuts and loosen the inner peels. Press on the chestnuts, through the towel, to force the slits to crack open. Remove and discard the shells and inner peels. You should get about 1 cup shelled chestnuts from 1/2 pound fresh chestnuts. To save time, substitute half (15-ounce) jar chopped roasted, peeled chestnuts or a 10-ounce can water-packed whole chestnuts, drained and chopped.

# Braised Chicken with Lentils and Gremolata

Typically served with osso buco, gremolata—a zesty mix of parsley, lemon, and garlic—adds pizzazz to this braised chicken. Complete the meal with steamed broccoli.

MAKES 4 SERVINGS

4 ($1/2$-pound) chicken legs, skin and fat removed
$1/2$ teaspoon salt
$1/2$ teaspoon ground pepper
2 teaspoons olive oil
1 large onion, chopped
2 celery ribs with leaves, chopped
1 large parsnip or carrot, chopped
1 (28-ounce) can Italian plum tomatoes
2 cups low-sodium chicken broth
1 cup lentils, picked over, rinsed, and drained
$1/4$ cup minced flat-leaf parsley
2 tablespoons grated lemon rind
2 large garlic cloves, minced

1. Sprinkle the chicken with the salt and pepper. Heat 1 teaspoon of the oil in a nonstick Dutch oven, then add the chicken. Cook over medium heat until lightly browned, about 3 minutes on each side. Transfer to a plate.
2. Heat the remaining 1 teaspoon oil in the same Dutch oven, then add the onion, celery, and parsnip or carrot. Cook over medium heat, stirring frequently, until softened, 3–4 minutes. Add the tomatoes, broth, lentils, and chicken; bring to a boil, stirring occasionally. Reduce the heat and simmer, covered, until the lentils are tender and the chicken is cooked through, 40–45 minutes.
3. To prepare the gremolata, combine the parsley, lemon rind, and garlic in a small bowl. Serve with the braised chicken.

■ PER SERVING (1 CHICKEN LEG AND ³/₄ CUP LENTILS): 483 calories, 12 g total fat, 3 g saturated fat, 87 mg cholesterol, 756 mg sodium, 51 g total carbohydrates, 16 g dietary fiber, 44 g protein, 148 mg calcium ■ *POINTS PER SERVING: 10*

*Tip:* Never discard celery leaves. They add great flavor to soups, stews, and braised dishes such as this. To remove the chicken skin easily, grasp the skin with a paper towel and gently pull; you'll find it comes off easily without slipping. Braising is a technique where the meat is first browned, then simmered in liquid until the meat gets very tender and falls easily from the bone. It's important to just simmer, not boil, the mixture.

# Paella

Now an American favorite, this classic Spanish meal-in-a-dish of chicken, shellfish, rice, saffron, and peas will fuel you with energy. If you own a two-handled, shallow paella pan, use it as the Spaniards do to cook and serve the paella. Otherwise cook the paella in a Dutch oven and serve it in a large shallow serving dish.

MAKES 6 SERVINGS

2 teaspoons olive oil
1/2 pound skinless boneless chicken breasts, cut into chunks
1 onion, chopped
2 garlic cloves, minced
2 1/4 cups low-sodium chicken broth
1 (14 1/2-ounce) can stewed tomatoes
1 1/4 cups long-grain white rice
1 red bell pepper, seeded and chopped
1/2 teaspoon ground pepper
1/8 teaspoon saffron threads
1/2 pound large shrimp, peeled and deveined
12 mussels, scrubbed and debearded
1 (10-ounce) package frozen peas
1 ounce thinly sliced prosciutto, cut into strips

1. Heat the oil in a nonstick Dutch oven, then add the chicken. Cook over medium-high heat until lightly browned on all sides, about 5 minutes. Transfer to a plate.
2. Add the onion and garlic to the same Dutch oven and cook over medium heat, stirring frequently, until softened, 3–5 minutes. Add the broth, tomatoes, rice, bell pepper, ground pepper, and saffron; bring to a boil. Reduce the heat and simmer, covered, until most of the liquid is absorbed and the rice is almost tender, about 15 minutes.
3. Stir in the shrimp, mussels, peas, prosciutto, and chicken. Cook, covered, until the shrimp are just opaque in the center, the mussels open, the chicken is cooked through, and the rice is tender, about 8 minutes. Discard any mussels that don't open.

■ PER SERVING (1 ½ CUPS): 325 calories, 5 g total fat, 1 g saturated fat, 69 mg cholesterol, 442 mg sodium, 46 g total carbohydrates, 4 g dietary fiber, 24 g protein, 73 mg calcium ■ *POINTS PER SERVING: 6*

*Tip:* The small amount of prosciutto adds a full, rich flavor to the paella. For the best flavor, choose prosciutto imported from Italy, such as prosciutto di Parma, also called Parma ham. After buying mussels, discard those with broken shells or shells that do not close tightly when tapped gently. Since mussels can be sandy, soak them in a bowl of cold water for 2–3 minutes. Repeat, using fresh water, until you can't see any more sand in the bowl. Then scrub them with a stiff brush under cold running water. To debeard mussels, pinch the hairy filaments that protrude from the shell between thumb and forefinger and pull firmly to remove.

# Lemon Chicken with Currant–Pine Nut Risotto

S weet currants and crunchy pine nuts give a welcome contrast of flavors and textures to this creamy risotto—a perfect accompaniment to the simple lemon chicken. Complete the meal with a green salad.

MAKES 4 SERVINGS

3 cups low-sodium chicken broth
1 tablespoon olive oil
1 onion, finely chopped
1 1/4 cups arborio rice
1/2 cup dry white wine
1/4 cup currants
1/4 cup pine nuts
1/4 cup chopped flat-leaf parsley
1/4 teaspoon ground pepper
4 (1/4-pound) skinless boneless chicken breasts
1 teaspoon grated lemon rind
1/2 teaspoon salt
4 lemon wedges

1. To prepare the risotto, bring the broth to a boil in a medium saucepan. Reduce the heat and keep at a simmer.
2. Heat the oil in a large nonstick saucepan, then add the onion. Cook over medium heat, stirring frequently, until softened, 3–5 minutes. Add the rice and cook until lightly toasted, 2–3 minutes.
3. Add the wine and 1/2 cup of the broth; cook, stirring until the liquid is absorbed. Continue to add the broth, 1/2 cup at a time, stirring until it is absorbed before adding more, until the rice is just tender and the mixture is creamy. (The cooking time from the first addition of broth should be 20–24 minutes.) Stir in the currants, pine nuts, parsley, and pepper.
4. Sprinkle the chicken with the lemon rind and salt. Spray a nonstick skillet with nonstick spray and set over medium heat. Add the chicken and cook until lightly browned

and just cooked through, about 5 minutes on each side. Transfer to a plate; let rest 5 minutes, then thinly slice on the diagonal. Serve with the risotto and lemon wedges.

■ PER SERVING (1 PIECE CHICKEN AND 1 CUP RISOTTO): 486 calories, 12 g total fat, 2 g saturated fat, 62 mg cholesterol, 403 mg sodium, 60 g total carbohydrates, 3 g dietary fiber, 33 g protein, 57 mg calcium ■ *POINTS PER SERVING: 10*

*Tip:* For perfect risotto every time, here are some simple guidelines: Use a short-grain rice, preferably arborio. Timing and temperature are key to successful risotto making. Be sure to keep the cooking broth just at a simmer on a nearby burner. Start counting total risotto cooking time from the first addition of broth. Cook the risotto over medium-low heat, or just enough heat to maintain a gentle simmer with each addition of liquid. Check the rice after 18–20 minutes of total cooking time. It should be tender and need an additional few minutes, at most.

# Jiffy Chicken Pepper Steak
# with Hash Browns

≡

**S**easoned pepper blend is a combination of coarsely ground black pepper and sweet bell peppers. It suffuses the chicken with spiciness and a touch of sweetness in this simple dish. Substitute a Szechuan-style pepper blend if you want to turn up the heat. You can find both in better supermarkets. A green salad tossed with apple slices makes a refreshing accompaniment.

### MAKES 4 SERVINGS

4 ($^{1}/_{4}$-pound) skinless boneless chicken breasts

1 teaspoon grated lime rind

2 tablespoons fresh lime juice

2 garlic cloves, minced

2 teaspoons canola oil

4 cups (from a 32-ounce bag) frozen hash brown potatoes

$^{1}/_{2}$ teaspoon salt

3 tablespoons chopped fresh parsley

2 tablespoons seasoned pepper blend (no salt added)

1. Place the chicken, lime rind, lime juice, and garlic in a large zip-close plastic bag; squeeze out the air and seal the bag; turn to coat the chicken. Let stand 10 minutes.

2. Meanwhile, heat the oil in a large nonstick skillet, then add the potatoes and salt. Cook, stirring frequently, until the potatoes are tender and lightly browned, about 10 minutes. Stir in the parsley.

3. Spread the pepper blend on wax paper. Remove the chicken from the marinade (discard the marinade) and lightly press into the pepper, coating both sides.

4. Spray a nonstick skillet or a nonstick ridged grill pan with nonstick spray and set over medium heat. Add the chicken and cook until it is lightly browned and just cooked through, 4–5 minutes on each side. Serve with the hash browns.

■ **PER SERVING (1 PIECE CHICKEN AND $^{3}/_{4}$ CUP HASH BROWNS):** 338 calories, 6 g total fat, 1 g saturated fat, 62 mg cholesterol, 400 mg sodium, 43 g total carbohydrates, 5 g dietary fiber, 28 g protein, 47 mg calcium ■ *POINTS PER SERVING: 6*

# Easy Chicken and Bean Enchiladas

Here's a meal the whole family will love. What's more, it's easy on the cook—a perfect dinner to whip up after you've been working late.

MAKES 4 SERVINGS

1 teaspoon canola oil
1 small onion, chopped
1 (15-ounce) can pinto beans, rinsed and drained
1 cup cubed cooked chicken breast
1 (14$^{1}/_{2}$-ounce) can diced tomatoes
1 (4-ounce) can chopped green chilis
$^{1}/_{4}$ cup chopped fresh cilantro
2 teaspoons chili powder
8 (6-inch) fat-free flour tortillas
$^{1}/_{2}$ cup shredded reduced-fat Monterey Jack cheese

1. Preheat the oven to 375° F. Spray a 7 × 11-inch baking dish with nonstick spray.
2. Heat the oil in a nonstick skillet, then add the onion. Cook over medium heat, stirring frequently, until golden, 7–10 minutes. Add the beans, chicken, $^{1}/_{2}$ cup of the tomatoes, the chilis, cilantro, and chili powder; cook until heated through, about 5 minutes.
3. Place about $^{1}/_{3}$ cup of the bean mixture onto each tortilla; roll up and place seam side down in the baking dish. Combine the remaining bean mixture (about $^{1}/_{3}$ cup) with the remaining tomatoes; spoon over the tortillas. Cover with foil and bake 20 minutes. Uncover and sprinkle with the cheese. Bake until heated through and the cheese is golden, about 8 minutes longer.

■ **PER SERVING (2 ENCHILADAS):** 371 calories, 6 g total fat, 3 g saturated fat, 34 mg cholesterol, 1,013 mg sodium, 54 g total carbohydrates, 10 g dietary fiber, 26 g protein, 240 mg calcium ■ *POINTS PER SERVING: 7*

*Tip:* If you like, you can substitute an equal amount of cooked, cubed pork loin for the chicken. To turn up the heat in this recipe, add a few drops of hot sauce to the tomatoes.

# Curried Turkey Cutlets

F ragrant Indian spices blended with yogurt transform ordinary turkey into something deliciously different. The marinade is also good for skinless, boneless chicken breasts or
lean pork cutlets. Serve with steamed potatoes, seasoned with chopped fresh mint, steamed
cauliflower and broccoli, and a spoonful of chutney.

## MAKES 4 SERVINGS

1 cup plain low-fat yogurt
4 garlic cloves, minced
2 tablespoons fresh lemon juice
2 tablespoons grated peeled fresh ginger
2 teaspoons ground cardamom
1 teaspoon ground cumin
3/4 teaspoon ground turmeric
1/2 teaspoon ground allspice
1/2 teaspoon salt
1/4 teaspoon cayenne
4 (1/4-pound) skinless boneless turkey cutlets
1/2 cup water
1 tablespoon chopped fresh mint

1. Place the yogurt, garlic, lemon juice, ginger, cardamom, cumin, turmeric, allspice,
   salt, and cayenne in a large zip-close plastic bag; squeeze the bag carefully to blend
   the ingredients. Add the turkey; squeeze out the air and seal the bag; turn to coat the
   turkey. Refrigerate, turning the bag occasionally, at least 1 hour or up to overnight.
2. Spray the broiler rack with nonstick spray; preheat the broiler.
3. Remove the turkey from the marinade. Reserve the marinade. Place the turkey on the
   broiler rack. Broil 5 inches from the heat until browned and just cooked though, 5–6
   minutes on each side.
4. Meanwhile, pour the marinade and the water into a small saucepan; bring to a boil.
   Boil, stirring occasionally, until the sauce thickens slightly, about 5 minutes. Spoon
   the sauce over the turkey and sprinkle with the mint.

■ PER SERVING (1 TURKEY CUTLET AND 2 TABLESPOONS SAUCE): 203 calories, 5 g total fat, 2 g saturated fat, 71 mg cholesterol, 401 mg sodium, 9 g total carbohydrates, 1 g dietary fiber, 30 g protein, 150 mg calcium ■ *POINTS PER SERVING: 4*

*Tip:* If a marinade for meat, poultry, or fish is to be used during cooking or as a sauce, it must be boiled at a rolling boil (that is, one that cannot be stirred down) for at least 3 minutes to kill any bacteria.

# Turkey and Spinach Lasagna Rolls

These unique cheese-and-spinach-stuffed lasagna bundles, smothered in a turkey marinara sauce, are easy to serve and delicious. They also provide built-in portion control.

MAKES 6 SERVINGS

6 lasagna noodles
1 teaspoon olive oil
$1/2$ pound ground skinless turkey breast
1 onion, chopped
1 yellow bell pepper, seeded and finely chopped
1 (16-ounce) container refrigerated fresh marinara sauce
$1/3$ cup water
1 cup nonfat ricotta cheese
$1/2$ (10-ounce) package frozen chopped spinach, thawed and squeezed dry
$1/4$ cup chopped fresh basil
2 tablespoons grated Parmesan cheese
1 large egg, lightly beaten
$1/8$ teaspoon ground nutmeg
$1/2$ cup shredded part-skim mozzarella cheese

1. Cook the lasagna noodles according to package directions. Drain and rinse the noodles and lay them flat on wax paper.

2. Heat the oil in a large nonstick skillet, then add the turkey, onion, and bell pepper. Cook, stirring frequently, until all the pan juices evaporate and the turkey browns, about 10 minutes. Stir in the marinara sauce and water; bring to a boil. Reduce the heat and simmer, uncovered, until slightly thickened and the flavors blend, about 5 minutes.

3. Preheat the oven to 375° F. Meanwhile, combine the ricotta cheese, spinach, basil, Parmesan cheese, egg, and nutmeg in a medium bowl. Spread the ricotta mixture over the length of each noodle and roll up from one short end.

4. Spread half of the turkey mixture in a 9-inch-square baking dish. Add the rolls. Top with the remaining turkey mixture. Cover with foil and bake 30 minutes. Remove the foil and sprinkle with the mozzarella. Bake until the top is golden, about 10 minutes.

■ **PER SERVING (1 ROLL WITH $1/6$ OF THE SAUCE):** 277 calories, 9 g total fat, 3 g saturated fat, 65 mg cholesterol, 496 mg sodium, 27 g total carbohydrates, 3 g dietary fiber, 23 g protein, 228 mg calcium ■ *POINTS PER SERVING: 6*

# Duck with Orange and Lime Sauce

Fresh duck is available from late spring to early winter. Or you can substitute skinless boneless turkey or chicken breasts, if you prefer.

MAKES 4 SERVINGS

4 (4-ounce) skinless, boneless duck breasts
1 teaspoon ground coriander
1/2 teaspoon salt
2 teaspoons canola oil
1 red onion, thinly sliced
1 jalapeño pepper, seeded and finely chopped (wear gloves to prevent irritation)
1/2 cup low-sodium chicken broth
1/2 cup orange juice
1 tablespoon honey
1 teaspoon grated lime rind
2 teaspoons lime juice
1 orange, sectioned
3 tablespoons chopped fresh cilantro
3 cups cooked jasmine rice

1. Sprinkle the duck with the coriander and salt. Heat 1 teaspoon of the oil in a large nonstick skillet, then add the duck. Cook over medium-high heat, until lightly browned, about 2 minutes on each side. Transfer the duck to a plate.

2. Heat the remaining 1 teaspoon oil in the same skillet, then add the onion and jalapeño pepper. Cook over medium-high heat, stirring frequently, until softened, 3–5 minutes. Add the broth, orange juice, honey, lime rind, lime juice, and duck; bring to a boil. Reduce the heat and simmer, covered, until the duck is cooked through, about 10 minutes. Transfer the duck to a serving platter. Bring the sauce to a rapid boil and boil until slightly thickened, 3–5 minutes.

3. Stir in the orange sections and the cilantro; heat through. Pour over the duck and serve with the rice.

■ **PER SERVING (1 PIECE DUCK WITH 1/4 CUP SAUCE AND 3/4 CUP RICE):** 414 calories, 12 g total fat, 4 g saturated fat, 73 mg cholesterol, 357 mg sodium, 49 g total carbohydrates, 2 g dietary fiber, 25 g protein, 55 mg calcium ■ *POINTS PER SERVING: 9*

# Fettuccine with Sausage and Arugula

A small amount of turkey sausage, a few beans, and some chicken broth seasoned with arugula, garlic, and fresh basil, make a light sauce for fettuccine. Toasted slices of Italian bread, topped with chopped roasted bell peppers, make a perfect accompaniment.

## MAKES 4 SERVINGS

1/2 pound whole-wheat fettuccine or other strand pasta

1/2 pound sweet turkey sausage

2 teaspoons extravirgin olive oil

1/4 pound fresh shiitake mushrooms, stems removed and sliced

1 small onion, chopped

3 garlic cloves, minced

1 (15-ounce) can cannellini (white kidney) beans, rinsed and drained

1 cup low-sodium chicken broth

5 ounces (4 cups lightly packed) arugula or spinach leaves

1 tomato, chopped

1/4 cup chopped fresh basil

1/4 teaspoon ground pepper

1. Cook the fettuccine according to package directions; drain.

2. Meanwhile, spray a large nonstick skillet with nonstick spray and set over medium-high heat. Add the sausage and brown, breaking it apart with a spoon, 3–4 minutes. Transfer to a plate.

3. Heat the oil in the same skillet, then add the mushrooms, onion, and garlic. Cook over medium heat, stirring frequently, until golden, 7–10 minutes. Add the beans, broth, arugula, and the browned sausage; bring to a boil. Reduce the heat and simmer, covered, until the sausage is cooked through and the arugula is just tender, about 3 minutes. Add the tomato, basil, and pepper; cook until just heated through, about 2 minutes. Serve with the fettuccine.

■ **PER SERVING (SCANT 1½ CUPS SAUSAGE MIXTURE AND 1 CUP FETTUCCINE):** 437 calories, 10 g total fat, 2 g saturated fat, 41 mg cholesterol, 835 mg sodium, 62 g total carbohydrates, 12 g dietary fiber, 28 g protein, 125 mg calcium ■
*POINTS PER SERVING: 9*

# Peppered Steak on Garlic Toast with Cherry Tomato Salsa

Tomatillos look like small green tomatoes and are covered with thin papery husks, which need to be removed. They have a firm flesh and a tart, lemony flavor. You can find them in the produce section of most supermarkets.

### MAKES 4 SERVINGS

6 whole unpeeled garlic cloves

3 cups water

1 pint grape or cherry tomatoes, halved

2 tomatillos, cut into small wedges

1/2 large seedless cucumber, peeled and diced

1/2 red onion, finely chopped

1/4 cup chopped fresh cilantro

1 jalapeño pepper, seeded and minced (wear gloves to prevent irritation)

3 tablespoons cider vinegar

1 tablespoon extravirgin olive oil

1/2 teaspoon salt

1 (1-pound) boneless beef sirloin steak

2 teaspoons dried oregano

1 teaspoon coarsely ground black pepper

4 (1-inch) slices seeded Italian bread, toasted

1. Bring the garlic and the water to a boil in a small saucepan. Reduce the heat and simmer, uncovered, until the garlic is very tender, about 15 minutes. Drain. When the garlic is cool enough to handle, remove the skins; put the garlic into a small bowl and mash. Set aside.
2. Spray the broiler rack with nonstick spray; preheat the broiler.
3. Meanwhile, to prepare the salsa, combine the tomatoes, tomatillos, cucumber, onion, cilantro, jalapeño, vinegar, oil, and salt in a medium bowl. Refrigerate, covered, until ready to serve.

4. Sprinkle the steak with the oregano and black pepper. Broil the steak 5 inches from the heat until done to taste, about 5 minutes on each side for medium. Let stand 10 minutes, then thinly slice the steak on an angle across the grain.

5. Spread the toast slices with the garlic puree. Arrange the meat on top of the bread slices. Top with the salsa. Serve at once.

> ■ **PER SERVING (¼ OF THE STEAK AND 1¼ CUPS SALSA):** 291 calories, 9 g total fat, 2 g saturated fat, 60 mg cholesterol, 521 mg sodium, 26 g total carbohydrates, 3 g dietary fiber, 27 g protein, 62 mg calcium ■ *POINTS PER SERVING: 6*

*Tip:* Poaching garlic is an easy way to mellow its strong taste—and it's a lot quicker and easier than roasting the garlic in the oven.

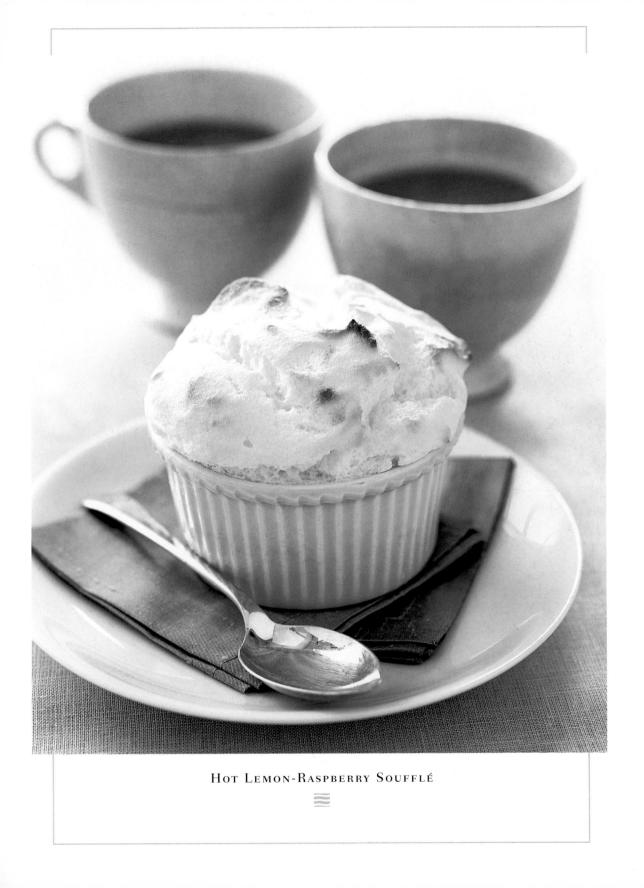

HOT LEMON-RASPBERRY SOUFFLÉ

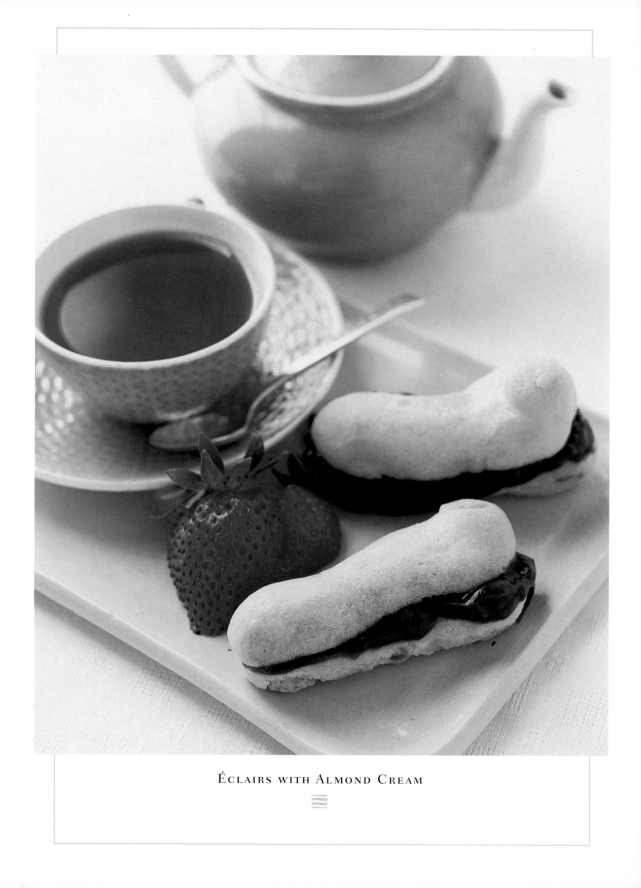

ÉCLAIRS WITH ALMOND CREAM

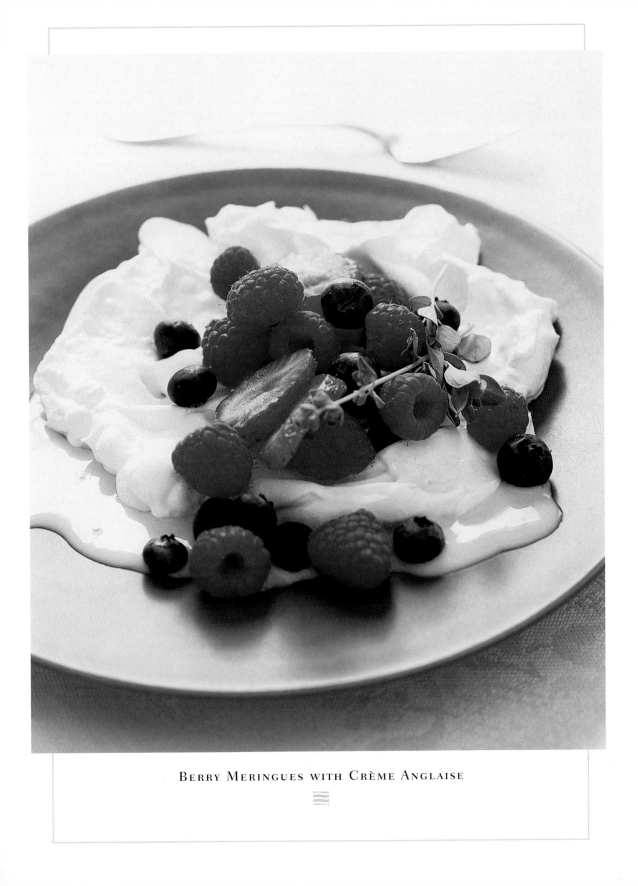

Berry Meringues with Crème Anglaise

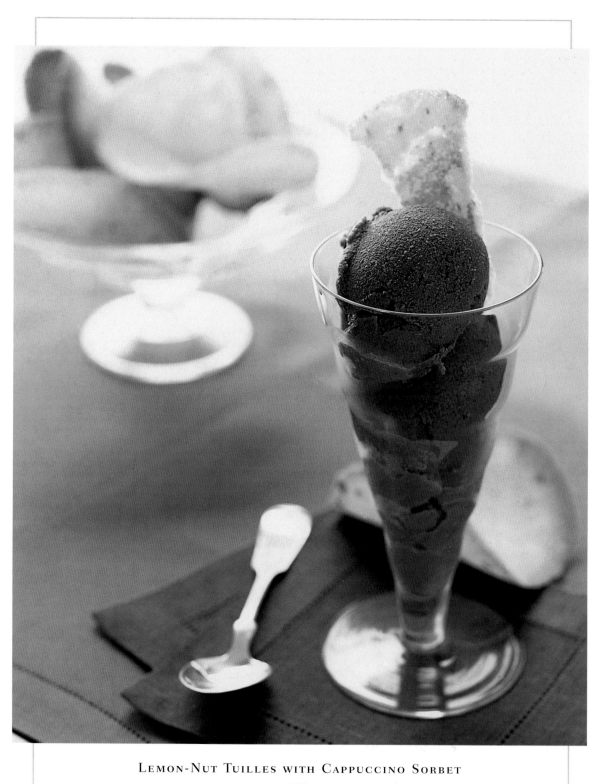

LEMON-NUT TUILLES WITH CAPPUCCINO SORBET

# Spicy Thai Beef Stir-Fry

Full of lively, robust flavors from watercress, lime juice, garlic, fresh ginger, and green curry paste, this spicy stir-fry will excite your taste buds. The fish sauce, Asian sesame oil, and green curry paste can be found in the gourmet section of your supermarket or in Asian markets. The curry sauce is quite hot, so a little goes a long way. If you can't find green curry paste, any hot chili paste will do.

MAKES 4 SERVINGS

3/4 cup low-sodium chicken broth
3 tablespoons fresh lime juice
3 tablespoons unsweetened coconut milk
2 tablespoons packed dark brown sugar
1 tablespoon cornstarch
1 tablespoon fish sauce (*nam pla*)
2 teaspoons Asian (dark) sesame oil
1/2 teaspoon green curry paste
2 teaspoons peanut oil
3/4 pound flank steak, cut across the grain diagonally into thin strips
2 garlic cloves, minced
1 teaspoon minced peeled fresh ginger
2 yellow bell peppers, seeded and cut into thin strips
1 bunch watercress (about 4 cups), tough stems removed
2 cups cooked brown rice

1. Combine the broth, lime juice, coconut milk, sugar, cornstarch, fish sauce, sesame oil, and curry paste in a bowl; set aside.
2. Heat a large nonstick skillet over high heat until a drop of water sizzles. Pour in 1 teaspoon of the peanut oil and swirl to coat the pan. Add the beef, in batches, and cook until browned, about 4 minutes. Transfer the beef to a plate. Wipe the skillet clean.
3. Heat the remaining 1 teaspoon peanut oil in the same skillet, then add the garlic and ginger. Stir-fry over medium-high heat, until fragrant, about 30 seconds. Add the peppers and cook, stirring constantly, until tender-crisp, about 3 minutes. Add the wa-

tercress and cook, stirring, until the watercress begins to wilt, about 3 minutes. Stir in the broth mixture and cook, stirring constantly, until the mixture boils and thickens, about 1 minute. Return the beef to the pan and toss to combine. Serve with the rice.

■ PER SERVING (1 1/2 CUPS STIR-FRY AND 1/2 CUP RICE): 366 calories, 14 g total fat, 5 g saturated fat, 48 mg cholesterol, 260 mg sodium, 37 g total carbohydrates, 3 g dietary fiber, 23 g protein, 74 mg calcium ■ *POINTS PER SERVING: 8*

# Orange Beef with Noodles

**H**ere's a classic Chinese favorite made so simple that you'll have dinner on the table in a mere 20 minutes.

MAKES 4 SERVINGS

4 ounces rice stick noodles

$2/3$ cup orange juice

2 tablespoons reduced-sodium soy sauce

2 teaspoons sugar

1 teaspoon Asian (dark) sesame oil

1 teaspoon cornstarch

$1/2$ teaspoon chili paste

$1/2$ pound flank steak, trimmed of all visible fat and sliced thin across the grain

6 scallions, cut into 2-inch slices

2 garlic cloves, minced

2 teaspoons peeled minced fresh ginger

1. Prepare the noodles according to package directions; drain.
2. Combine the orange juice, soy sauce, sugar, oil, cornstarch, and chili paste in a bowl until blended and smooth; set aside.
3. Spray a large nonstick skillet with nonstick spray and set over high heat. Add the steak and cook in batches, until browned, about 5 minutes. Add the scallions, garlic, and ginger. Cook, stirring constantly, until fragrant, about 3 minutes. Stir in the orange juice mixture and cook until the sauce boils and thickens slightly, about 3 minutes. Stir in the noodles; heat through. Serve at once.

■ **PER SERVING (1¼ CUPS):** 210 calories, 5 g total fat, 2 g saturated fat, 32 mg cholesterol, 342 mg sodium, 26 g total carbohydrates, 1 g dietary fiber, 14 g protein, 34 mg calcium ■ *POINTS PER SERVING: 4*

*Tip:* When browning meat, make sure it is cooked over high heat in a single layer. If your pan is not big enough to accommodate all the meat at one time, cook it in batches, otherwise the meat will steam instead of brown.

# Bolognese Sauce with Fettuccine

≡

**B**olognese, a hearty meat sauce from the northern Italian city of Bologna, is given a wonderful earthy flavor by dried porcini mushrooms and fresh white mushrooms. This sauce is also great in lasagna or spooned over chunky shaped pasta such as rigatoni, ziti, or tortellini.

### MAKES 4 SERVINGS

1/2 cup dried porcini mushrooms
1 cup hot water
1 tablespoon olive oil
2 carrots, finely chopped
1 onion, finely chopped
1 rib celery, finely chopped
1/2 pound sliced white mushrooms
1/2 pound lean ground beef (10% or less fat)
1 cup dry white wine
1/2 cup low-fat (1%) milk
1/8 teaspoon ground nutmeg
1 (28-ounce) can Italian peeled tomatoes, drained and chopped
3/4 teaspoon salt
3 tablespoons fat-free half-and-half
3 tablespoons chopped fresh parsley
8 ounces fettuccine

1. Combine the porcini mushrooms and the hot water in a small bowl; let stand 20 minutes to soften. Drain the mushrooms, reserving their liquid. Coarsely chop the mushrooms.
2. Heat the oil in a large nonstick saucepan, then add the carrots, onion, and celery. Cook over medium-high heat, stirring occasionally, until the vegetables are very soft, about 8 minutes. Add the porcini and the sliced mushrooms. Cook, stirring occasionally, until the mushrooms are soft, about 5 minutes. Add the beef and cook, breaking up the pieces with a fork, until the meat is no longer pink, about 6 minutes. Drain and discard any remaining fat.

3. Stir in the wine and bring to a boil. Reduce the heat and simmer, uncovered, until the wine has evaporated, about 10 minutes. Add the milk and nutmeg; simmer, stirring frequently, until the milk has evaporated, about 5 minutes.

4. Stir in the reserved mushroom liquid, the tomatoes, and the salt; bring to a boil. Reduce the heat and simmer, covered, until the flavors are blended and the sauce has thickened, about 1 hour. Stir in the half-and-half and parsley. Remove from the heat.

5. Cook the fettuccine according to package directions; drain. Transfer the pasta and sauce to a large bowl; toss to coat.

■ PER SERVING (1 3/4 CUPS): 424 calories, 11 g total fat, 3 g saturated fat, 83 mg cholesterol, 760 mg sodium, 56 g total carbohydrates, 6 g dietary fiber, 25 g protein, 152 mg calcium ■ *POINTS PER SERVING: 9*

# Lemon Veal Chops with
# Tomato and Olive Couscous

The fragrant lemon-parsley rub gives excellent flavor to the veal, while the couscous adds a boost of carbohydrate energy. This rub also tastes delicious on chicken or pork.

2 teaspoons olive oil

1 tomato, chopped

1 tablespoon minced shallot

1 (10-ounce) box plain couscous

2 cups low-sodium chicken broth

4 oil-cured black olives, pitted and chopped

1 tablespoon chopped fresh parsley

2 teaspoons dried oregano

2 teaspoons grated lemon rind

1 garlic clove, minced

$1/2$ teaspoon salt

$1/2$ teaspoon ground pepper

4 (6-ounce) lean, bone-in veal chops, about $1/2$-inch thick, trimmed of all visible fat

1. Spray the broiler rack with nonstick spray; preheat the broiler.
2. Heat 1 teaspoon of the oil in a medium nonstick saucepan, then add the tomato and shallot. Cook over medium heat until the tomato is softened, about 4 minutes. Add the couscous, broth, and olives; bring to a boil. Remove from the heat; let stand, covered, 5 minutes. Fluff lightly with a fork.
3. Meanwhile, combine the parsley, oregano, lemon rind, garlic, salt, pepper, and the remaining 1 teaspoon oil in a small bowl. Blot the veal chops dry with paper towels. Rub both sides of the veal with the parsley mixture. Broil 5 inches from the heat until done to taste, 3–4 minutes on each side for medium-rare. Serve with the couscous.

■ **PER SERVING (1 VEAL CHOP AND 3/4 CUP COUSCOUS):** 408 calories, 7 g total fat, 2 g saturated fat, 62 mg cholesterol, 417 mg sodium, 58 g total carbohydrates, 4 g dietary fiber, 26 g protein, 54 mg calcium ■ *POINTS PER SERVING: 8*

# Braised Veal with Mushroom Risotto

**T**here's nothing like braising to bring out the best flavor of tough cuts of meat such as veal shanks. In braising, the meat is first browned to seal in the juices, then simmered for a long time to develop the flavors. Make sure to have a tight-fitting lid to prevent the liquid from evaporating. If you like, substitute lamb shanks for the veal.

MAKES 6 SERVINGS

1 teaspoon olive oil
4 (7-ounce) veal shanks, trimmed of all fat
1 carrot, chopped
1 onion, finely chopped
1 celery rib, chopped
$1/2$ teaspoon dried thyme
$3^1/4$ cups low-sodium chicken broth
1 (16-ounce) can Italian peeled tomatoes, drained and chopped
$1/4$ cup dry white wine
1 bay leaf
3 cups water
1 teaspoon olive oil
1 cup sliced mushrooms
$1^1/3$ cups arborio rice
$1/2$ teaspoon salt
$1/2$ teaspoon ground pepper
$1/4$ cup grated Parmesan cheese

1. Preheat the oven to 350° F.
2. Heat a flameproof 3–quart casserole dish or nonstick Dutch oven over high heat. Swirl in the oil, then add the veal shanks and cook until lightly browned, about 3 minutes on each side. Transfer to a plate.
3. To the same casserole dish, add the carrot, half of the onion, the celery, and the thyme. Cook over medium heat, stirring frequently, until golden, 7–10 minutes.
4. Stir in 2 cups of the broth, the tomatoes, wine, and bay leaf; bring to a boil. Add the veal and spoon some of the vegetables over the shanks. Cover the casserole and place

it in the oven. Braise until the veal is fork-tender, about 1 1/2 hours. Skim and discard any fat on the surface of the sauce.

5. Prepare the risotto 30 minutes before the veal is done: Bring the water and the remaining 1 1/4 cups broth to a boil in a medium saucepan. Reduce the heat and keep at a simmer.

6. Heat the oil in a large nonstick saucepan, then add the mushrooms and the remaining half of the onion. Cook over medium heat, stirring occasionally, until very tender, about 8 minutes. Add the rice and cook, stirring, until lightly toasted, about 4 minutes. Add 1 cup of the broth mixture and stir until the liquid is absorbed.

7. Continue to add the broth, 1/2 cup at a time, stirring until it is absorbed before adding more, until the rice is just tender and the mixture is creamy. The cooking time from the first addition of broth should be 20–24 minutes. Stir in the salt, pepper, and cheese.

8. Remove the veal from the casserole and remove the meat from the bones. Discard the bay leaf and bones. Return the veal to the sauce and serve with the risotto.

■ PER SERVING (1 1/4 CUPS VEAL WITH SAUCE AND 2/3 CUP RISOTTO): 406 calories, 10 g total fat, 4 g saturated fat, 115 mg cholesterol, 495 mg sodium, 42 g total carbohydrates, 2 g dietary fiber, 34 g protein, 132 mg calcium ■ *POINTS PER SERVING: 9*

# Roast Pork Tenderloin with Apple Glaze and Maple Mashed Potatoes

P ork tenderloin is the fillet of pork. It is as lean as skinless, boneless chicken breasts and when cooked properly is very moist and tender.

MAKES 4 SERVINGS

3 sweet potatoes, peeled and quartered
1 tablespoon apple jelly
1 tablespoon chopped fresh thyme
1 garlic clove, minced
1 teaspoon salt
$^1/_2$ teaspoon coarsely ground black pepper
1 (1-pound) boneless pork tenderloin, trimmed of all fat
3 tablespoons maple syrup
3 tablespoons packed brown sugar
$^1/_8$ teaspoon ground nutmeg

1. Preheat the oven to 475° F. Spray a shallow roasting pan with nonstick spray.
2. Place the potatoes and enough water to cover in a large saucepan; bring to a boil. Reduce the heat and simmer, covered, until the potatoes are tender, about 20 minutes; drain.
3. Meanwhile, combine the apple jelly, thyme, garlic, $^1/_2$ teaspoon of the salt, and the pepper in a small bowl. Rub the jelly mixture all over the pork.
4. Spray a large nonstick skillet with nonstick spray and set over high heat. Add the pork and sear until brown on all sides, about 8 minutes. Transfer to the roasting pan and roast until an instant-read thermometer, inserted into the thickest part of the pork, registers 160° F., about 20 minutes. Let stand 10 minutes before slicing.
5. Transfer the potatoes to a mixing bowl. Add the maple syrup, sugar, remaining $^1/_2$ teaspoon salt and nutmeg; beat with an electric mixer on medium speed, until blended.
6. Slice the pork diagonally into $^1/_4$-inch thick slices and serve with the sweet potatoes.

■ **PER SERVING ($^1/_4$ OF THE PORK AND $^1/_2$ CUP POTATOES):** 319 calories, 4 g total fat, 1 g saturated fat, 67 mg cholesterol, 645 mg sodium, 44 g total carbohydrates, 3 g dietary fiber, 26 g protein, 54 mg calcium ■ *POINTS PER SERVING: 6*

# Thai Curry Pork Kebabs

romatic basmati rice is a perfect accompaniment to these spicy kebabs. For a change, try the curry sauce with grilled salmon or chicken.

### MAKES 4 SERVINGS

2/3 cup basmati rice

1/2 cup unsweetened coconut milk

3 tablespoons packed dark brown sugar

1 tablespoon reduced-sodium soy sauce

2 teaspoons minced peeled fresh ginger

1 garlic clove, minced

1/2 teaspoon red curry paste

2 teaspoons curry powder

1 teaspoon paprika

1/2 teaspoon ground cumin

2 tablespoons chopped fresh cilantro

1 pound boneless pork tenderloin, trimmed of all fat and cut into 1 1/2-inch cubes

1 tablespoon unsalted dry-roasted peanuts, chopped

1. Cook the rice according to the package directions; keep warm.
2. Spray the broiler rack with nonstick spray; preheat the broiler.
3. Whisk together the coconut milk, brown sugar, soy sauce, ginger, garlic, and red curry paste in a small bowl. Place the curry powder, paprika, and cumin in a dry skillet over low heat. Cook, shaking the pan and stirring constantly, until fragrant, 1–2 minutes. Whisk in the coconut mixture and bring to a boil; boil 1 minute. Remove from the heat and stir in 1 tablespoon of the cilantro; reserve 1/4 cup of the sauce for serving.
4. Thread the pork onto four 10-inch metal skewers. Brush the pork with the remaining sauce. Broil the kebabs 5 inches from the heat, until cooked, about 12 minutes.
5. Spoon the rice onto a large platter. Top with the kebabs. Drizzle the kebabs and rice with the reserved 1/4 cup sauce. Sprinkle with the peanuts and the remaining 1 tablespoon cilantro.

■ **PER SERVING (1 KEBAB AND 1/2 CUP RICE):** 387 calories, 12 g total fat, 7 g saturated fat, 67 mg cholesterol, 216 mg sodium, 40 g total carbohydrates, 1 g dietary fiber, 28 g protein, 42 mg calcium ■ *POINTS PER SERVING: 9*

# Country-Style Lamb and Barley Stew

S tews are often better the next day, when the spices have mingled and the flavors have had a chance to develop—and this recipe is no exception. If you make it a day ahead and refrigerate it, the stew will be rich and robust by the time you serve it.

MAKES 6 SERVINGS

1 teaspoon olive oil
1 pound lean lamb cubes for stew
1 onion, chopped
2 garlic cloves, minced
1 tablespoon tomato paste
1 tablespoon chopped fresh rosemary
6 cups low-sodium chicken broth
1/2 cup pearl barley, rinsed
2 carrots, cut into 1/4-inch slices
1/2 pound green beans, trimmed and cut into 1-inch pieces
1 (9-ounce) package frozen pearl onions
1 cup frozen peas

1. Heat the oil in a large nonstick saucepan, then add the lamb. Cook over medium-high heat until browned on all sides, about 6 minutes. Add the onion and garlic. Cook, stirring frequently, until the onion is softened, about 5 minutes. Stir in the tomato paste and rosemary until blended. Add the broth and barley; bring to a boil. Reduce the heat and simmer, covered, until the lamb and barley are tender, about 40 minutes.

2. Add the carrots, beans, and pearl onions. Simmer, uncovered, until the vegetables are tender, about 6 minutes. Stir in the peas; heat through.

   ■ **PER SERVING (1 1/3 CUPS):** 245 calories, 6 g total fat, 2 g saturated fat, 42 mg cholesterol, 143 mg sodium, 28 g total carbohydrates, 7 g dietary fiber, 20 g protein, 61 mg calcium ■ *POINTS PER SERVING: 5*

# Moroccan Stuffed Eggplant

This mild, sweet filling includes golden raisins and pine nuts—also called pignoli. Pine nuts have a delicate flavor and are used in many sweet and savory dishes of the Mediterranean.

MAKES 4 SERVINGS

2 small (12- to 14-ounce) eggplants, halved lengthwise
1 teaspoon olive oil
$1/2$ pound lean ground lamb (10% or less fat)
1 small tomato, chopped
1 onion, finely chopped
1 garlic clove, minced
$1/4$ cup plain dry bread crumbs
$1/4$ cup golden raisins
1 tablespoon pine nuts, toasted
1 large egg, lightly beaten
$1/2$ teaspoon salt
$1/4$ teaspoon ground allspice

1. Preheat the oven to 400° F. Spray a shallow baking dish with nonstick spray.
2. Bring a large pot of water to a boil. Add the eggplant, cut side down. Reduce the heat and simmer, covered, until the eggplant is just tender, about 5 minutes. Drain the eggplant on paper towels; let cool.
3. Meanwhile, heat the oil in a nonstick skillet, then add the lamb, tomato, onion, and garlic. Cook over medium-high heat, stirring occasionally, until the lamb is no longer pink, about 6 minutes. Transfer the mixture to a bowl.
4. Carefully scoop out the pulp from each eggplant half with a spoon, leaving a $1/4$-inch thick shell. Coarsely chop the pulp.
5. Mix the eggplant pulp with the lamb mixture, the bread crumbs, raisins, pine nuts, egg, salt, and allspice. Spoon the filling into the eggplant shells and place in the baking dish. Bake until the filling is heated through and browned on top, 25 minutes.

■ PER SERVING (¹/₂ STUFFED EGGPLANT): 247 calories, 8 g total fat, 2 g saturated fat, 94 mg cholesterol, 406 mg sodium, 27 g total carbohydrates, 6 g dietary fiber, 17 g protein, 48 mg calcium ■ *POINTS PER SERVING: 5*

*Tip:* Like all nuts, pine nuts should be stored in the freezer to prevent them from turning rancid.

# Spiced Tuna with Red Pepper Pesto

T una steaks are perfect for pan-searing. Make sure they are at least 3/4-inch thick, because if they are cut too thin, the center of the tuna will dry out before the outside has had a chance to form a golden crust. The robust pesto is also delicious tossed with your favorite pasta or spread on toasted Italian bread for a quick snack or appetizer.

### MAKES 4 SERVINGS

2 red bell peppers
1/2 cup fresh basil leaves
5 kalamata olives, pitted
2 garlic cloves
1 shallot, halved
1 tablespoon pine nuts, toasted
2 tablespoons fennel seeds, very finely chopped
1 tablespoon chopped fresh thyme
1 teaspoon extravirgin olive oil
1/4 teaspoon salt
1/4 teaspoon ground pepper
4 (6-ounce) tuna steaks, 3/4-inch thick

1. Preheat the broiler. Line a baking sheet with foil; place the peppers on the baking sheet. Broil 5 inches from the heat, turning frequently with tongs, until the skin is lightly charred on all sides, about 10 minutes. Place the peppers in a medium bowl, cover with plastic wrap, and let steam 10 minutes. When cool enough to handle, peel, seed, and coarsely chop; set aside.

2. Purée the peppers, basil, olives, garlic, shallot, and pine nuts in a blender or food processor. Transfer the pesto to a bowl.

3. Combine the fennel seeds, thyme, oil, salt, and pepper. Rub both sides of the tuna steaks with the fennel mixture.

4. Spray a nonstick skillet with nonstick spray and set over medium heat. Add the tuna and cook until browned on the outside but still pink in the center, about 3 minutes on each side. Drizzle the pesto over the tuna.

■ **PER SERVING (1 TUNA STEAK AND ¼ CUP PESTO):** 299 calories, 12 g total fat, 3 g saturated fat, 65 mg cholesterol, 259 mg sodium, 6 g total carbohydrates, 2 g dietary fiber, 41 g protein, 62 mg calcium ■ *POINTS PER SERVING: 7*

*Tip:* Spray the fennel seeds with nonstick spray before chopping to prevent them from scattering over the cutting board.

# Salmon Persillade with Horseradish Mashed Potatoes

P ersillade, a sprightly combination of parsley and garlic, is mixed with bread crumbs and lemon to make a delicious crunchy topping for salmon. To round out the meal, serve a vitamin- and mineral-rich green vegetable, such as steamed broccoli.

### MAKES 4 SERVINGS

8 cups water
1 pound red potatoes, peeled and quartered
1 pound salmon fillet, cut into 4 pieces
4 teaspoons Dijon mustard
1/4 cup plain dry bread crumbs
1 tablespoon chopped fresh parsley
1 garlic clove, minced
2 teaspoons grated lemon rind
1 teaspoon olive oil
3/4 teaspoon salt
1/3 cup low-fat (1%) milk
3 tablespoons light sour cream
2 tablespoons prepared horseradish
Fresh parsley sprigs

1. Bring the water and potatoes to a boil in a large saucepan. Reduce the heat and simmer, covered, until the potatoes are fork-tender, about 20 minutes. Drain and keep warm.

2. Preheat the oven to 425° F. Spray a baking sheet with nonstick spray. Place the salmon on the baking sheet; brush the tops with the mustard.

3. Combine the bread crumbs, parsley, garlic, lemon rind, oil, and 1/4 teaspoon of the salt in a bowl. Sprinkle the bread crumb mixture on top of the salmon; spray lightly with nonstick spray. Bake until the salmon is just opaque in the center and the topping is golden brown, about 15 minutes.

4.  Meanwhile, transfer the potatoes to a large bowl; add the milk, sour cream, horse-radish, and the remaining $1/2$ teaspoon salt. Beat with an electric mixer on medium speed until the potatoes are smooth and creamy. Serve with the salmon and garnish with the parsley sprigs.

    ▨ **PER SERVING (1 PIECE SALMON AND** $1/2$ **CUP POTATOES):** 318 calories, 9 g total fat, 3 g saturated fat, 79 mg cholesterol, 662 mg sodium, 29 g total carbohy-drates, 2 g dietary fiber, 29 g protein, 90 mg calcium ▨ *POINTS PER SERVING: 7*

# Flounder en Papillote

G et a lot of flavor without a lot of fat by cooking foods en papillote, or in a parchment paper parcel. The parchment puffs up as the food cooks and will surely impress guests. For less glorious occasions, use foil instead of parchment paper.

MAKES 4 SERVINGS

1 teaspoon olive oil
1 large carrot, cut into matchstick-thin strips
1 leek, white part only, cleaned and thinly sliced
1 tomato, chopped
1 tablespoon chopped fresh thyme
1 garlic clove, minced
$1/4$ teaspoon salt
4 (4-ounce) flounder fillets
$1/4$ cup dry white wine

1. Heat the oil in a nonstick skillet, then add the carrot, leek, tomato, thyme, garlic, and salt. Cook over medium-low heat, stirring frequently, until the vegetables are very tender, about 10 minutes. Remove from the heat; set aside.
2. Preheat the oven to 425° F. Fold four 12 × 16-inch sheets parchment paper in half. Starting at the folded edge, cut each paper into a half heart shape. Unfold and spray the parchment paper with nonstick spray.
3. Arrange the fish on half of each piece of parchment. Top with the vegetable mixture. Sprinkle with the wine. Fold the parchment over the fish and vegetables, into packets, making a tight seal. Place the parchment parcels on a baking sheet and bake until they are puffy and the flounder is opaque in the center, about 8 minutes.

■ **PER SERVING (1 PARCEL):** 132 calories, 3 g total fat, 0 g saturated fat, 56 mg cholesterol, 247 mg sodium, 6 g total carbohydrates, 2 g dietary fiber, 21 g protein, 37 mg calcium ■ *POINTS PER SERVING: 2*

*Tip:* Parchment parcels are traditionally made in heart shapes, but you can use 14-inch squares of parchment. Fill them, gather the edges to make a pouch, and tie the neck with string.

# Cajun Fish and Sweet Potato Chips

 **A** Cajun twist on an old British favorite makes this fish spicy and the potato "chips" sweet, crispy, and simply irresistible.

### MAKES 4 SERVINGS

2 large sweet potatoes, unpeeled and cut into rounds, $^1/_4$-inch thick

1 tablespoon olive oil

$^1/_4$ teaspoon salt

$^1/_4$ cup reduced-calorie mayonnaise

2 tablespoons sweet pickle relish

1 teaspoon Dijon mustard

1 pound catfish fillets, cut into 4 pieces

1 tablespoon Cajun seasoning

1. Preheat the oven to 400° F.
2. Combine the potatoes with $2^1/_2$ teaspoons of the olive oil and the salt in a large bowl until well coated. Spread the potatoes in one layer on a wire rack placed on a baking sheet. Bake until crisp, about 30 minutes.
3. Meanwhile, to prepare the tartar sauce, combine the mayonnaise, relish, and mustard in a small bowl. Refrigerate, covered, until ready to serve.
4. Sprinkle the fish with the Cajun seasoning. Heat the remaining $^1/_2$ teaspoon oil in a large nonstick skillet, then add the fish. Cook over medium-high heat until the fish is just opaque in the center, about 3 minutes on each side. Serve with the sweet potato chips and the tartar sauce.

■ **PER SERVING (1 PIECE CATFISH WITH 1$^1/_2$ TABLESPOONS TARTAR SAUCE AND 3/4 CUP CHIPS):** 302 calories, 10 g total fat, 2 g saturated fat, 74 mg cholesterol, 831 mg sodium, 26 g total carbohydrates, 4 g dietary fiber, 26 g protein, 50 mg calcium ■ *POINTS PER SERVING: 6*

*Tip:* For easy cleanup, line the baking sheet for the chips with foil.

# Lemon Cod with Spinach and Potato Stew

This one-skillet dish of seared cod, simmered in a light stew of potatoes and fresh spinach with a hint of lemon, boasts a complex, delicious flavor. Yet it's so simple to make, it's a perfect weeknight stand-by recipe.

### MAKES 4 SERVINGS

1 pound cod fillet, cut into 4 pieces
$1/2$ teaspoon salt
$1/4$ teaspoon ground pepper
1 tablespoon olive oil
1 onion, thinly sliced
1 garlic clove, minced
1 tomato, chopped
1 pound red potatoes, unpeeled, scrubbed, and quartered
$2^1/2$ cups low-sodium chicken broth
2 teaspoons grated lemon rind
1 tablespoon fresh lemon juice
2 tablespoons cold water
1 tablespoon all-purpose flour
$1/2$ (10-ounce) bag fresh baby spinach, cleaned

1. Sprinkle both sides of the cod with the salt and pepper. Heat 1 teaspoon of the oil in a large nonstick skillet, then add the cod. Cook over medium-high heat until the cod is just opaque in the center and browned on the outside, about 3 minutes on each side. Transfer to a plate; set aside.

2. Heat the remaining 2 teaspoons oil in the same skillet, then add the onion and garlic. Cook over medium-low heat, stirring occasionally, until the onion is very tender, about 8 minutes. Add the tomato; cook until soft, about 5 minutes. Add the potatoes, broth, lemon rind, and lemon juice; bring to a boil. Reduce the heat and simmer, covered, until the potatoes are fork-tender, about 15 minutes.

3.  Meanwhile, whisk together the water and flour in a small bowl until smooth. Stir into the simmering vegetables. Add the spinach. Cook, stirring constantly, until the sauce thickens and the spinach begins to wilt, 2–3 minutes. Return the cod to the skillet; heat through.

■ **PER SERVING (1 PIECE COD AND 1¼ CUPS STEW):** 282 calories, 6 g total fat, 1 g saturated fat, 60 mg cholesterol, 459 mg sodium, 31 g total carbohydrates, 4 g dietary fiber, 27 g protein, 77 mg calcium ■ *POINTS PER SERVING: 5*

# Baked Sea Bass
# with Fennel and Olives

≡

The aromatic flavors of fennel, olives, and orange truly complement the sea bass in this simple, yet delicious, entrée. If you don't like the anise flavor of fennel, you can substitute 2 cups of thinly sliced celery instead. A good substitute for the bass would be red snapper or cod fillets.

### MAKES 4 SERVINGS

1 tablespoon olive oil

$1/2$ fennel bulb, thinly sliced

1 onion, thinly sliced

1 garlic clove, minced

3 plum tomatoes, chopped

6 kalamata olives, pitted and coarsely chopped

1 tablespoon grated orange rind

$1/2$ cup fresh chopped basil

4 ($1/4$ pound) sea bass fillets

$1/2$ teaspoon salt

$1/4$ teaspoon ground pepper

1. Preheat the oven to 400° F. Spray a nonstick 9 × 13-inch baking dish with nonstick spray.

2. Heat the oil in a large nonstick skillet, then add the fennel, onion, and garlic. Cook over medium-high heat, stirring frequently, until golden, 7–10 minutes. Stir in the tomatoes, olives, and orange rind. Cook until the tomatoes begin to soften, about 5 minutes. Remove from the heat; stir in the basil.

3. Sprinkle the fish with the salt and pepper. Place the fish skin side down in the baking dish. Spoon the fennel mixture on top. Cover with foil and bake until the fish is just opaque in the center, about 25 minutes.

■ **PER SERVING:** 173 calories, 6 g total fat, 1 g saturated fat, 60 mg cholesterol, 456 mg sodium, 8 g total carbohydrates, 2 g dietary fiber, 23 g protein, 54 mg calcium ■ *POINTS PER SERVING: 4*

# Monkfish, Cajun Style

≡

**M**onkfish, sometimes called angler fish, is a low-fat, firm-textured fish with a mild, sweet taste. We've spiked the flavor with Cajun seasoning and a garlicky tomato sauce. Cooked brown rice makes a perfect accompaniment to this dish.

MAKES 4 SERVINGS

1 pound monkfish fillets, cut into 4 pieces
2 tablespoons Cajun seasoning
1 tablespoon olive oil
2 green bell peppers, seeded and thinly sliced
1 large onion, thinly sliced
2 garlic cloves, minced
1 (14$\frac{1}{2}$-ounce) can stewed tomatoes
1 tablespoon chopped fresh thyme or 1 teaspoon dried

1. Sprinkle the fish with 1 tablespoon of the Cajun seasoning. Heat 1 teaspoon of the oil in a large nonstick skillet, then add the fish. Cook over medium-high heat until browned, about 3 minutes on each side. Transfer the fish to a plate; set aside.
2. Heat the remaining 2 teaspoons oil in the same skillet, then add the peppers, onion, garlic, and the remaining 1 tablespoon Cajun seasoning. Cook over medium heat, stirring occasionally, until the vegetables are very tender, about 8 minutes. Add the tomatoes with their liquid and the thyme; bring to a boil. Return the monkfish to the skillet. Reduce the heat and simmer, covered, until the flavors are blended and the fish is opaque in the center, about 8 minutes.

■ **PER SERVING (1 MONKFISH FILLET AND 1 CUP SAUCE):** 196 calories, 5 g total fat, 1 g saturated fat, 62 mg cholesterol, 1,144 mg sodium, 14 g total carbohydrates, 2 g dietary fiber, 24 g protein, 65 mg calcium ■ *POINTS PER SERVING: 4*

≡

# Garlicky Shrimp Scampi

**S**poon the scampi over parsleyed rice or noodles and serve with lemon wedges. Complete the meal with a side salad of baby Boston lettuce and thin red bell pepper strips.

### MAKES 4 SERVINGS

1 tablespoon olive oil
1 pound large shrimp, peeled, deveined, and butterflied
3 garlic cloves, minced
$1/4$ teaspoon salt
$1/4$ teaspoon ground pepper
$1/2$ cup dry white wine
$1/2$ cup low-sodium chicken broth
2 tablespoons fresh lemon juice
3 scallions, sliced
2 tablespoons chopped fresh parsley
$1/3$ cup plain dry bread crumbs

1. Preheat the broiler.
2. Heat the oil in a large nonstick ovenproof skillet, then add the shrimp, garlic, salt, and pepper. Cook over medium-high heat, stirring occasionally, until the shrimp begin to turn pink, about 3 minutes. Add the wine, broth, lemon juice, scallions, and parsley; bring to a boil. Reduce the heat and simmer, uncovered, until the liquid begins to thicken slightly and the shrimp are just opaque, about 3 minutes.
3. Top the shrimp mixture with the bread crumbs and place the skillet under the broiler 4 inches from the heat. Broil until the topping is golden, about 3 minutes.

■ **PER SERVING (1 1/4 CUPS):** 137 calories, 5 g total fat, 1 g saturated fat, 107 mg cholesterol, 359 mg sodium, 9 g total carbohydrates, 1 g dietary fiber, 13 g protein, 61 mg calcium ■ *POINTS: 3.*

*Tip:* To butterfly shrimp, peel the shrimp. Then, using a paring knife, slice along the back of the shrimp from top to tail, cutting the shrimp almost but not entirely in half. With the blade of your knife, scrape out the vein and flatten the shrimp slightly.

# Creamy Fettuccine
# with Scallops and Spinach

For a nice variation and a pretty color contrast, try this with carrot or tomato fettuccine instead of plain fettuccine. To give an extra energy boost, serve with thin breadsticks such as grissini—add one point for every two breadsticks.

### MAKES 4 SERVINGS

1/2 pound fettuccine

2 tablespoons all-purpose flour

1/2 teaspoon salt

1/4 teaspoon ground nutmeg

2 cups low-fat (1%) milk

2 teaspoons olive oil

3/4 pound sea scallops, patted dry and muscle tabs removed

6 ounces portobello mushrooms, sliced (about 2 cups)

1 shallot, finely chopped

1 tablespoon reduced-sodium soy sauce

2 pounds spinach, cleaned and coarsely chopped

1. Cook the fettuccine according to the package directions. Drain; keep warm.
2. Combine the flour, salt, and nutmeg in a medium nonstick saucepan. Gradually whisk in the milk and cook over medium heat, stirring constantly, until the sauce boils and thickens, about 8 minutes. Remove the white sauce from the heat; set aside.
3. Meanwhile, heat 1 teaspoon of the oil in a large nonstick skillet, then add the scallops. Cook over medium-high heat until lightly browned on the outside and just opaque in the center, about 2 minutes on each side. Transfer the scallops to a plate. Wipe the skillet clean.
4. Heat the remaining 1 teaspoon oil in the same skillet, then add the mushrooms, shallot, and soy sauce. Cook over medium heat, stirring occasionally, until the mushrooms are tender and browned, about 5 minutes. Stir in the fettuccine, white sauce, scallops, and spinach, tossing to coat well. Cook, stirring frequently, until the mixture is heated through and the spinach just wilts, about 4 minutes.

■ **PER SERVING (1 ½ CUPS):** 431 calories, 8 g total fat, 2 g saturated fat, 81 mg cholesterol, 870 mg sodium, 57 g total carbohydrates, 7 g dietary fiber, 36 g protein, 436 mg calcium ■ *POINTS PER SERVING: 8*

*Tip:* I suggest taking a few extra minutes to nip off the too-tough-to-chew muscle tabs attached to sea scallops before cooking them. To get the scallops to brown around the edges, make sure they are patted thoroughly dry with paper towels before you sauté them.

# Mussels with Garlic, Tomatoes, and Wine

One scent of these mussels in their aromatic broth, and you'll be transported to a little fishing village in the Mediterranean. Serve with crusty bread to sop up the juices.

MAKES 4 SERVINGS

1 tablespoon olive oil
3 shallots, thinly sliced
3 garlic cloves, minced
1 tablespoon chopped fresh thyme
6 plum tomatoes, chopped
2 pounds mussels, scrubbed and debearded
1 1/2 cups low-sodium chicken broth
1/2 cup dry white wine
1/4 cup chopped fresh basil

1. Heat the oil in a large nonstick saucepan, then add the shallots, garlic, and thyme. Cook over medium heat, stirring occasionally, until the shallots are softened, about 3 minutes. Add the tomatoes and cook until soft and the flavors are blended, about 8 minutes. Stir in the mussels, broth, and wine; bring to a boil, stirring occasionally. Reduce the heat and simmer, covered, until the mussels have opened, about 5 minutes. Discard any mussels that do not open.

2. Transfer the mussels to four bowls; stir the basil into the broth, then pour over the mussels.

■ PER SERVING: 148 calories, 5 g total fat, 1 g saturated fat, 34 mg cholesterol, 92 mg sodium, 10 g total carbohydrates, 2 g dietary fiber, 15 g protein, 81 mg calcium ■ *POINTS PER SERVING: 3*

*Tip:* When purchasing mussels, look for unbroken, tightly closed shells or shells that close when lightly tapped. Scrub them with a stiff brush under running cold water to remove any sand. Discard any shells that remain open. The hairy filaments that protrude from a mussel are known as a "beard." To remove, pinch the filaments between thumb and forefinger and pull firmly.

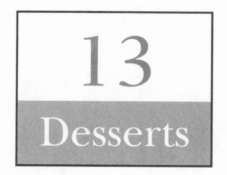

# Desserts

## Lemon Angel Food Cake

This delicate cake is delicious all on its own, but for a truly impressive dessert, spoon orange segments and raspberries on top. Serve with cappuccino made with fat-free milk.

**MAKES 12 SERVINGS**

2 cups sifted cake flour (not self-rising)
12 egg whites
1 1/4 teaspoons cream of tartar
2 cups sugar
1 tablespoon grated lemon rind
1 teaspoon lemon extract
Confectioners' sugar for dusting

1. Preheat the oven to 375° F. Sift the flour into a small bowl; set aside.
2. With an electric mixer at medium speed, beat the egg whites and cream of tartar in a large bowl until thick and foamy. Gradually sprinkle in the sugar and continue beating until the egg whites form medium peaks, 3–5 minutes.
3. With a large spatula, fold in the flour in 3 additions, gently folding each addition into the egg whites until well combined. Fold in the lemon rind and lemon extract.
4. Pour the batter into an ungreased 10-inch tube pan. Bake until the cake springs back when touched lightly, 35–40 minutes. Invert the cake in the pan onto its legs or onto a bottle; cool completely in the pan.

5. To serve, carefully loosen the cake from the pan with a metal spatula; place on a cake plate, bottom-side up and sprinkle with the confectioners' sugar.

▪ PER SERVING (1/12 CAKE): 219 calories, 0 g total fat, 0 g saturated fat, 0 mg cholesterol, 56 mg sodium, 49 g total carbohydrates, 0 g dietary fiber, 5 g protein, 121 mg calcium ▪ *POINTS PER SERVING: 4*

*Tip:* Be sure to use a serrated knife when slicing the cake, wiping the blade with a damp towel each time you slice. The tube pan used to make this dessert should be absolutely clean and grease free. Any residue in the pan will prevent the cake from rising properly.

# Fresh Peach Cake

Y ou'll want to use the juiciest peaches you can find for this lovely dessert. If peaches are not in season, you can substitute 6 cups of thawed frozen sliced peaches. Just make sure to drain them well and pat dry with paper towels. Fresh nectarines, plums, and apricots also make an excellent choice.

MAKES 12 SERVINGS

2 1/4 cups reduced-fat baking mix
7 tablespoons sugar
2/3 cup low-fat (1%) milk
3 tablespoons melted butter
8 (about 2 pounds) ripe peaches, pitted and sliced (6 cups)
3/4 cup light nondairy whipped topping

1. Preheat the oven to 425° F. Spray an 8-inch-square cake pan with nonstick spray. Line the bottom of the cake pan with wax paper. Spray the wax paper with nonstick spray.
2. Combine the baking mix, 5 tablespoons of the sugar, the milk, and the butter in a medium bowl until blended. Scrape the dough into the pan.
3. Bake until a toothpick inserted in the center comes out clean, 20–25 minutes. Cool the cake in the pan on a rack 10 minutes; remove from the pan and cool completely on the rack.
4. Toss the peaches with the remaining 2 tablespoons sugar in a bowl until the sugar dissolves. Split the cooled cake in half horizontally. Place the bottom layer onto a cake plate; top with half of the peach mixture. Spoon the whipped topping over the peaches. Place the remaining cake layer on top. Spoon the remaining peaches into the center. Serve immediately.

■ PER SERVING (1/12 CAKE): 177 calories, 5 g total fat, 3 g saturated fat, 8 mg cholesterol, 275 mg sodium, 30 g total carbohydrates, 2 g dietary fiber, 3 g protein, 42 mg calcium ■ *POINTS PER SERVING: 4*

# Raspberry Cheesecake

D on't worry if your cake cracks: cracking is characteristic of cheesecakes after they are baked, especially when using nonfat ingredients. However, spooning fresh berries on top hides the cracking and makes for a beautiful presentation. This cheesecake is better made a day, or even two days, ahead and kept in the refrigerator.

10 reduced-fat cinnamon graham crackers
2 tablespoons applesauce
1 tablespoon melted butter
4 (8-ounce) packages nonfat cream cheese
1 1/4 cups sugar
1 cup fat-free egg substitute
1 tablespoon fresh lemon juice
1 teaspoon vanilla extract
1 pint fresh raspberries
Confectioners' sugar for dusting

1. Preheat the oven to 350° F. Spray a 9-inch springform pan with nonstick spray.
2. Place the graham crackers in a large zip-close plastic bag. Crush the crackers with a rolling pin until fine crumbs form. Transfer the crumbs to a bowl. Stir in the applesauce and butter until blended. Scatter the crumb mixture evenly over the bottom of the pan. Refrigerate the pan until ready to use.
3. With an electric mixer at medium speed, beat the cream cheese in a large bowl until smooth. Gradually beat in the sugar until well blended. Beat in the egg substitute, lemon juice, and vanilla extract until combined. Pour the filling evenly onto the crust.
4. Bake the cheesecake until a knife inserted in the center comes out clean, 45–50 minutes. Cool completely on a rack. Refrigerate, covered, at least 12 hours or up to 3 days before serving.
5. To serve, remove the sides of the pan. Top the cheesecake with the raspberries, then sprinkle with confectioners' sugar.

■ **PER SERVING (1/12 CHEESECAKE):** 218 calories, 2 g total fat, 1 g saturated fat, 4 mg cholesterol, 462 mg sodium, 36 g total carbohydrates, 2 g dietary fiber, 13 g protein, 94 mg calcium ■ *POINTS PER SERVING: 4*

# Hot Lemon-Raspberry Soufflé

Individual hot lemon soufflés with a raspberry surprise on the bottom make a light, refreshing finish to any meal. If you don't own soufflé molds, use 6-ounce custard cups.

MAKES 6 SERVINGS

2 tablespoons plus $1/3$ cup sugar
$1/4$ cup seedless raspberry jam
1 tablespoon butter
3 tablespoons all-purpose flour
$2/3$ cup low-fat (1%) milk
1 tablespoon grated lemon rind
$1/2$ cup fresh lemon juice
2 egg yolks
4 egg whites
Confectioners' sugar for dusting

1. Preheat the oven to 400° F. Spray six 6-ounce soufflé molds with nonstick spray. Sprinkle 2 tablespoons of the sugar into one of the molds, turning constantly, so the sugar coats the bottom and sides. Toss the sugar remaining in the mold into the next mold, and repeat until all the molds are coated. Spoon 1 teaspoon raspberry jam into the bottom of each mold. Refrigerate the molds until ready to use.

2. Heat the butter in a small nonstick saucepan until melted. Sprinkle in the flour and whisk until smooth. Cook over low heat, stirring constantly, 1 minute. Whisk in the milk and bring to a boil, whisking constantly. Remove from heat and transfer the milk mixture to a bowl. Stir in the lemon rind and lemon juice. Stir in the egg yolks, one at a time, until blended.

3. With an electric mixer at medium speed, beat the egg whites in a medium bowl until soft peaks form, 2–3 minutes. Sprinkle in the remaining $1/3$ cup sugar; continue beating until stiff, glossy peaks form, about 3 minutes. Stir about $1/4$ of the beaten egg whites into the milk mixture to lighten. With a rubber spatula, gently fold in the remaining egg whites.

4. Spoon the batter into the soufflé molds, filling each about three-quarters full. Arrange the molds in a roasting pan, lined with paper towels to prevent them from slipping. Place the pan in the oven, then carefully fill the roasting pan with hot water until it reaches two-thirds up the sides of the soufflé molds. Bake until golden brown and puffed, about 25 minutes. Carefully remove the soufflés from the water bath. Dust with confectioners' sugar and serve at once.

■ **PER SERVING (1 SOUFFLÉ):** 170 calories, 4 g total fat, 2 g saturated fat, 77 mg cholesterol, 76 mg sodium, 30 g total carbohydrates, 0 g dietary fiber, 5 g protein, 49 mg calcium ■ *POINTS PER SERVING: 4*

*Tip:* For extra-light, high-volume soufflés, have the egg whites at room temperature and make sure the bowl and beater you use to beat the egg whites are squeaky clean.

# Blueberry Clafouti

≡

lafouti is a light, custardlike French dessert. It can be made with a variety of fresh fruits or berries. Substitute pitted ripe cherries, sliced peaches, pears, or apples for the blueberries if you prefer.

Makes 8 servings

4 cups blueberries
$^1\!/_2$ cup low-fat (1%) milk
$^1\!/_2$ cup sugar
3 tablespoons all-purpose flour
2 large eggs
1 tablespoon melted butter
2 teaspoons grated lemon rind
$^1\!/_2$ teaspoon ground cinnamon
Confectioners' sugar for dusting

1. Preheat the oven to 375° F. Spray a shallow 2–quart baking dish with nonstick spray. Spoon the blueberries into the baking dish.
2. Process the milk, sugar, flour, eggs, butter, lemon rind, and cinnamon in a food processor until smooth. Pour the batter over the berries.
3. Bake, uncovered, until the top is golden and a knife inserted in the center comes out clean, 35–40 minutes. Cool to room temperature on a rack, about 1 hour. Sprinkle with the confectioners' sugar just before serving.

■ **PER SERVING ($^1\!/_8$ CLAFOUTI):** 139 calories, 3 g total fat, 1 g saturated fat, 58 mg cholesterol, 38 mg sodium, 26 g total carbohydrates, 2 g dietary fiber, 3 g protein, 32 mg calcium ■ *POINTS PER SERVING: 3*

≡

# Coeur à la Crème with Apricot Sauce

This light, creamy French dessert is traditionally made in ceramic heart-shaped molds with perforated bottoms to allow any moisture to drain. However, this lighter version needs no special molds. Simply line individual custard cups with dampened cheesecloth to make unmolding easier. Coeur à la crème can be made up to a day ahead and refrigerated.

MAKES 4 SERVINGS

6 ounces nonfat cream cheese
1/4 cup confectioners' sugar
1 teaspoon vanilla extract
3/4 cup light nondairy whipped topping
3/4 cup apricot jam
1/4 cup water
1 teaspoon fresh lemon juice
Fresh mint sprigs

1. With an electric mixer at high speed, beat the cream cheese, sugar, and vanilla in a medium bowl until blended. Gently fold in the whipped topping.
2. Cut a sheet of cheesecloth into four 8-inch squares and dampen slightly with cold water. Line four 6-ounce custard cups with the cheesecloth, allowing the excess to overhang. Spoon the cream cheese mixture into the custard cups. Fold the excess cheesecloth over the tops. Refrigerate until just set, about 2 hours or overnight.
3. Bring the jam, water, and lemon juice to a boil in a small saucepan. Cook, stirring constantly, until the mixture melts and thickens slightly, about 3 minutes; let cool. Refrigerate, covered, until ready to use.
4. To serve, invert the molds onto individual plates and peel off the cheesecloth. Serve with the apricot sauce and the mint sprigs.

■ PER SERVING (1 COEUR À LA CRÈME AND 3 TABLESPOONS APRICOT SAUCE): 240 calories, 2 g total fat, 1 g saturated fat, 1 mg cholesterol, 238 mg sodium, 51 g total carbohydrates, 1 g dietary fiber, 7 g protein, 67 mg calcium ■
*POINTS PER SERVING: 5*

# Éclairs with Almond Cream

É clairs, made from cream puff dough—also known as choux pastry or pâte à choux— are much easier to make than you think. If you like, fill them with prepared, sugar-free pudding or light nondairy whipped topping instead of making the almond cream.

### CREAM PUFF DOUGH
1 cup water
$^1/_4$ cup butter
1 teaspoon granulated sugar
$^1/_8$ teaspoon salt
1 cup all-purpose flour
1 large egg
2 egg whites

### ALMOND CREAM
$^1/_4$ cup granulated sugar
2 tablespoons all-purpose flour
$^1/_2$ teaspoon salt
$1^1/_2$ cups low-fat (1%) milk
1 large egg
1 teaspoon almond extract
Confectioners' sugar for dusting

1. Preheat the oven to 400° F. Lightly spray a large baking sheet with nonstick spray. Line the baking sheet with parchment paper.
2. To make the cream puff dough, bring the water, butter, sugar, and salt to a boil in a medium saucepan. Stir in the flour all at once; cook, stirring constantly with a wooden spoon, until the dough begins to pull away from the sides of the pan, 1–2 minutes. Remove from the heat and stir in the egg and egg whites, one at a time, beating vigorously after each addition, until the dough is shiny and smooth. The dough will separate as you add the eggs, but with continued beating it will smooth out, become stiff, and hold its shape.

3. Spoon the dough into a pastry bag fitted with a $1/2$-inch plain tip. Pipe the dough onto the baking sheet into twelve $31/2$-inch strips. Bake until golden, about 30 minutes. Let rest on the baking sheet until cool enough to handle, 2–3 minutes, then split in half lengthwise with a sharp knife to allow the steam to escape. Remove and discard some of the soft dough from the centers. Cool the éclairs completely on a rack.

4. To prepare the Almond Cream, combine the sugar, flour, and salt in a medium saucepan. Whisk in the milk and egg. Cook over medium-low heat, stirring constantly, until the mixture coats the back of a spoon, about 8 minutes (do not boil, or the mixture may curdle). Remove from the heat, then stir in the almond extract. Transfer to a small bowl.

5. Place the bowl into a larger bowl filled with ice cubes and water. Refrigerate, covered, until the mixture mounds when dropped from a spoon, about 30 minutes.

6. Spoon about 2 tablespoons of the pastry cream into each éclair. Dust with confectioners' sugar and serve at once.

■ **PER SERVING (1 ÉCLAIR):** 128 calories, 5 g total fat, 3 g saturated fat, 47 mg cholesterol, 133 mg sodium, 16 g total carbohydrates, 0 g dietary fiber, 4 g protein, 45 mg calcium ■ *POINTS PER SERVING: 3*

*Tip:* To dust with confectioners' sugar, place about 1 to 2 tablespoons confectioners' sugar in a small sieve and sift over the éclairs.

# Berry Meringues
# with Crème Anglaise

≡

Meringues—light, delicious, and fat free! What could be better? Here, they are topped with fresh berries and served with a light crème anglaise (custard sauce). For a change, top them with low-fat ice cream, frozen yogurt, or fresh fruit.

MAKES 8 SERVINGS

4 egg whites
1/4 teaspoon cream of tartar
3/4 cup plus 1/3 cup granulated sugar
13/4 cups low-fat (1%) milk
1 vanilla bean, halved lengthwise or 1 teaspoon pure vanilla extract
3 egg yolks
1 cup fresh strawberries, hulled and sliced
1 cup fresh blueberries
1 cup fresh raspberries
Confectioners' sugar for dusting

1. Preheat the oven to 200° F. Line 2 large baking sheets with foil.
2. With an electric mixer at medium speed, beat the egg whites and the cream of tartar in a large bowl just until frothy. Gradually sprinkle in 3/4 cup of the sugar, 2 tablespoons at a time, until the sugar completely dissolves and the whites stand in stiff, glossy peaks, about 8 minutes.
3. Spoon the egg white mixture onto the baking sheets, making eight 6-inch rounds. Spread the mixture with the back of a spoon or a small metal spatula, leaving about 1/2 inch between the meringues.
4. Bake the meringues until they feel crisp to the touch, about 2 hours. Turn the oven off and leave the meringues in the oven until they are crisp and dry to the touch, about 1 hour longer.
5. Cool the meringues on the baking sheets on racks 10 minutes. Carefully loosen and transfer the meringues with a metal spatula to the rack to cool completely.

6. Meanwhile, to prepare the crème anglaise, bring the milk and vanilla bean to a boil in a medium saucepan; remove from the heat. Remove the vanilla bean, scraping the fragrant seeds from inside the bean into the milk. If using vanilla extract, stir it into the hot milk mixture off the heat.

7. Meanwhile, whisk the egg yolks and the remaining $1/3$ cup sugar in a bowl until the sugar is dissolved and the mixture is slightly thickened and pale yellow. Whisk $1/2$ cup of the hot milk mixture into the egg mixture. Slowly pour the egg mixture back into the hot milk mixture, whisking quickly and constantly. Cook over low heat, stirring constantly, until the mixture thickens and coats the back of a spoon, about 6 minutes. Do not boil, or the mixture may curdle. Transfer the custard to a bowl; let cool. Refrigerate, covered, until chilled at least 2 hours, or up to 2 days.

8. To serve, combine the strawberries, blueberries, and raspberries in a bowl. Drizzle about 3 tablespoons of the crème anglaise onto each serving plate. Top each plate with a meringue, then about $1/3$ cup of the berries and a sprinkling of confectioners' sugar.

■ PER SERVING (1 MERINGUE, $1/3$ CUP BERRIES, AND 3 TABLESPOONS CRÈME ANGLAISE): 184 calories, 3 g total fat, 1 g saturated fat, 82 mg cholesterol, 59 mg sodium, 36 g total carbohydrates, 2 g dietary fiber, 5 g protein, 83 mg calcium ■ *POINTS PER SERVING: 4*

*Tip:* Humidity can play a factor in the crispness of meringues, so don't make them on a rainy or humid day.

# Lemon-Nut Tuiles

≡

Tuiles (pronounced tweel), French for "tiles," are thin, crisp cookies that resemble the shape of a curved roof tile. While still warm and just out of the oven, they are draped over a rolling pin to create their characteristic curved shape. Serve these cookies with low-fat frozen yogurt or fresh berries. They are also delicious on their own with a cup of freshly brewed coffee.

MAKES 12 SERVINGS

$^1\!/_2$ cup sugar
3 tablespoons butter
$^1\!/_2$ teaspoon almond extract
2 egg whites
1 tablespoon grated lemon rind
$^1\!/_3$ cup all-purpose flour
$^1\!/_4$ cup sliced almonds, coarsely chopped

1. Preheat the oven to 400° F. Spray a large baking sheet with nonstick spray. Line with parchment paper.
2. Pulse the sugar, butter, and almond extract in a food processor until just mixed, about 20 seconds. Add the egg whites and lemon rind; pulse until just blended, about 15 seconds longer. Add the flour and process just until blended, about 10 seconds. Transfer the mixture to a bowl; stir in the almonds.
3. Working in batches, drop rounded tablespoonfuls of the batter onto the baking sheet. Spread the batter out very thinly with the back of a spoon into 4-inch rounds, about 1 inch apart. You will get about 4 cookies on each sheet.
4. Bake until the cookies are lightly browned and the edges are dry, about 10 minutes. Cool on the baking sheet about 1 minute. Then, using a small knife or metal spatula, lift the cookies and place them over a rolling pin to give them a curved shape until set, about 10 minutes. Repeat with the remaining batter, making a total of 12 cookies. Store the cookies in an airtight container for up to 3 days.

■ PER SERVING (1 COOKIE): 85 calories, 4 g total fat, 2 g saturated fat, 8 mg cholesterol, 29 mg sodium, 12 g total carbohydrates, 0 g dietary fiber, 1 g protein, 7 mg calcium ■ *POINTS PER SERVING: 2*

# Orange-Berry Crêpes with Ricotta Cream

≡

R eminiscent of Crêpes Suzette, these crêpes make an elegant yet substantial brunch. The berries add delicious flavor (not to mention a good dose of fiber, vitamins, and minerals), and the orange-scented ricotta adds an appealing creamy contrast (and a touch of protein and calcium).

1 cup fat-free milk
2 large eggs
1 cup all-purpose flour
2 teaspoons canola oil
1/4 teaspoon salt
1 cup part-skim ricotta cheese
2 tablespoons confectioners' sugar
3 tablespoons orange juice
3 teaspoons grated orange rind
2 cups fresh blueberries
1 cup fresh raspberries
2 tablespoon packed light brown sugar
1 tablespoon orange liqueur or vanilla extract
2 tablespoons toasted sliced almonds

1. To make the crêpes, beat the milk, eggs, flour, oil, and salt in a medium bowl until smooth; let stand at least 15 minutes.
2. Spray a crêpe pan or 6-inch nonstick skillet with nonstick spray; heat over medium-high heat until a drop of water sizzles. Pour in 2 tablespoons of the batter and swirl to cover the pan. Cook until the underside is set, about 30 seconds. Flip and cook until lightly browned, about 1 minute longer. Slide the crêpe onto wax paper. Repeat with the remaining batter, making a total of 12 crêpes; stack the crêpes between sheets of wax paper to prevent them from sticking to each other.
3. To make the ricotta cream, combine the ricotta cheese, confectioners' sugar, 2 tablespoons of the orange juice, and 1 teaspoon of the orange rind in a small bowl.

4. Combine the blueberries, raspberries, brown sugar, liqueur, and the remaining 1 tablespoon orange juice and 2 teaspoons orange rind in a large skillet; bring to a boil. Reduce the heat and simmer, uncovered, until slightly thickened, about 2 minutes. Fold the crêpes into quarters and place in the sauce. Simmer until the crêpes are hot, turning them once in the sauce, about 2 minutes. Serve with the ricotta cream and sprinkle with the almonds.

   ■ PER SERVING (3 CRÊPES WITH ¼ OF THE SAUCE AND ¼ CUP RICOTTA CREAM): 408 calories, 12 g total fat, 4 g saturated fat, 126 mg cholesterol, 293 mg sodium, 58 g total carbohydrates, 5 g dietary fiber, 17 g protein, 286 mg calcium ■ *POINTS PER SERVING: 8*

   *Tip:* To toast the almonds, place them in a small dry skillet over medium-low heat. Cook, shaking the pan and stirring constantly, until lightly browned and fragrant, 3–4 minutes. Watch them carefully when toasting; almonds can burn quickly. Transfer the nuts to a plate to cool.

# Banana Cream Crêpes with Chocolate Sauce

≡

These thin, delicate pancakes can be served with a variety of fillings and are perfect for brunch. If you like, substitute your favorite berries or peaches or nectarines for the bananas. Or simply spread them with jam and sprinkle with confectioners' sugar.

MAKES 4 SERVINGS

1/2 cup low-fat (1%) milk
1/4 cup all-purpose flour
1 large egg
2 teaspoons sugar
Pinch of salt
2 ripe bananas, thinly sliced
1 tablespoon chopped toasted pecans
1/2 teaspoon ground cinnamon
3/4 cup light nondairy whipped topping
1/4 cup bottled chocolate sauce

1. To make the crêpes, beat the milk, flour, egg, sugar, and salt in a medium bowl until smooth; let stand at least 15 minutes.
2. Meanwhile, combine the bananas, pecans, and cinnamon in a bowl. Gently fold in the whipped topping until just blended.
3. Spray a crêpe pan or 6-inch nonstick skillet with nonstick spray; heat over medium-high heat until a drop of water sizzles. Pour in one-fourth of the batter and swirl to cover the pan. Cook until the underside is set, about 30 seconds. Flip and cook until lightly browned, about 1 minute longer. Slide the crêpe onto wax paper. Repeat with the remaining batter, making a total of 4 crêpes; stack the crepes between sheets of wax paper to prevent them from sticking to each other.
4. Top each crêpe with 1/4 of the banana mixture; roll to enclose the filling. Drizzle with the chocolate sauce. Repeat with the remaining crêpes, filling, and sauce.

■ PER SERVING (1 FILLED CRÊPE AND 1 TABLESPOON CHOCOLATE SAUCE): 201 calories, 5 g total fat, 2 g saturated fat, 55 mg cholesterol, 129 mg sodium, 38 g total carbohydrates, 2 g dietary fiber, 5 g protein, 64 mg calcium ■ *POINTS PER SERVING: 4*

*Tip:* If you want to have extra crepes on hand, double the batter. Layer the extras between sheets of wax paper, place in a food storage bag, and freeze for up to 3 months. The batter can be made up to a day ahead and refrigerated. Be sure to let the batter stand at least 15 minutes before cooking in order to give the flour time to absorb the liquid.

# Summer Fruit and Ginger Shortcake

A generous portion of peaches, nectarines, plums, and kiwi fruit, sparkling with fresh mint, makes a healthy topping for low-fat ginger shortcake. For an extra 2 points per serving, top with 1/2 cup fat-free frozen yogurt.

MAKES 6 SERVINGS

2 1/4 cups reduced-fat baking mix
5 tablespoons sugar
2 tablespoons chopped candied ginger
2/3 cup low-fat (1%) milk
3 tablespoons reduced-calorie margarine, melted
2 peaches, sliced
2 nectarines, sliced
2 plums, sliced
2 kiwi fruit, peeled and cut into chunks
3 tablespoons orange juice
1 tablespoon chopped fresh mint
Mint sprigs (optional)

1.  Preheat the oven to 425° F. Spray a 9-inch pie dish with nonstick spray.
2.  Combine the baking mix, 3 tablespoons of the sugar, the ginger, milk, and margarine in a medium bowl until blended. Scrape the batter into the pie plate.
3.  Bake until a toothpick inserted in the center comes out clean, 20–25 minutes. Cool in the pie dish on a rack 5 minutes; remove from the pie dish and cool 10 minutes on the rack.
4.  Meanwhile, combine the peaches, nectarines, plums, kiwi fruit, orange juice, the remaining 2 tablespoons sugar, and the mint in a large bowl. Cut the shortcake into wedges, spoon the fruit mixture over each wedge. Garnish with mint sprigs (if using).

■ **PER SERVING (1/6 SHORTBREAD AND 2/3 CUP FRUIT):** 322 calories, 7 g total fat, 1 g saturated fat, 1 mg cholesterol, 587 mg sodium, 60 g total carbohydrates, 3 g dietary fiber, 6 g protein, 89 mg calcium ■ *POINTS PER SERVING: 6*

*Tip:* Before chopping the candied ginger, spray the knife with nonstick spray to keep the ginger from sticking to the knife as you chop.

# Strawberry-Orange Sorbet

**K**eep this sorbet covered in the freezer for up to 1 month and take out $^{1}/_{2}$ cup at a time for a refreshing treat.

MAKES 6 SERVINGS

4 cups strawberries, hulled and rinsed
$^{1}/_{2}$ cup frozen orange juice concentrate
$^{1}/_{3}$ cup sugar
2 tablespoons orange liqueur

Purée the strawberries, orange juice, sugar, and liqueur in a food processor or blender. Pour into an 8-inch-square baking dish and freeze until the mixture is frozen 1 inch around the edges, about $1^{1}/_{2}$ hours. Stir the mixture well to break up the large crystals. Return to the freezer and freeze until firm, at least 2 hours.

■ **PER SERVING ($^{1}/_{2}$ CUP):** 104 calories, 0 g total fat, 0 g saturated fat, 0 mg cholesterol, 1 mg sodium, 24 g total carbohydrates, 2 g dietary fiber, 1 g protein, 17 mg calcium ■ *POINTS PER SERVING: 2*

# Cappuccino Sorbet

Easy to make (no ice-cream machine required), this sorbet will give you an energy boost on the hottest of days. Partially frozen in a shallow pan and whirled to a creamy smooth consistency in a food processor, it's a cinch to make.

MAKES 8 SERVINGS

3 cups water
1 cup sugar
3/4 cup unsweetened cocoa powder
1/2 cup light corn syrup
2 (1-ounce) squares, semisweet chocolate, chopped
1 tablespoon instant espresso powder
1 teaspoon ground cinnamon
1/4 teaspoon ground nutmeg
1 cup fat-free half-and-half

1. Bring the water, sugar, cocoa powder, corn syrup, chocolate, espresso, cinnamon, and nutmeg to a boil in a saucepan. Reduce the heat and simmer until the sugar dissolves, about 5 minutes. Remove from the heat. Stir in the half-and-half. Pour into a 9 × 13-inch baking dish. Cover with plastic wrap and freeze until partially frozen, about 2 hours.
2. Working in batches, spoon the sorbet into a food processor or blender. Process 1 minute. Pour back into the baking dish. Cover with plastic wrap and freeze 1 hour.
3. Repeat step 2. Freeze until firm, about 1 1/2 hours.

■ PER SERVING (1/2 CUP): 228 calories, 3 g total fat, 2 g saturated fat, 0 mg cholesterol, 52 mg sodium, 53 g total carbohydrates, 3 g dietary fiber, 3 g protein, 58 mg calcium ■ *POINTS PER SERVING: 4*

# 14

## Bonus! Snappy Snacks

## White Pizza Muffins

W hen you want pizza in a hurry, English muffins are the way to go. Be as creative as you like with the toppings: use leftovers, such as chicken, turkey, or cooked broccoli pieces, instead of the turkey ham.

### MAKES 4 SERVINGS

1/2 cup nonfat ricotta cheese
2 English muffins, split and toasted
1/2 cup low-fat turkey ham, chopped
1/2 cup shredded part-skim mozzarella cheese

Preheat the broiler. Spread the ricotta cheese on the muffin halves. Top with the turkey ham and sprinkle with the mozzarella cheese. Place the pizzas on the broiler rack and broil, 4 inches from the heat, until the cheese is melted and bubbly, about 4 minutes.

■ PER SERVING (1 MUFFIN HALF): 154 calories, 4 g total fat, 2 g saturated fat, 12 mg cholesterol, 402 mg sodium, 16 g total carbohydrates, 1 g dietary fiber, 13 g protein, 204 mg calcium ■ *POINTS PER SERVING: 3*

# Smoked Salmon Melba Toasts

Instant energy—and elegance. Substitute thinly sliced prosciutto ham for the smoked salmon, if you prefer.

### MAKES 1 SERVING

1 tablespoon light cream cheese (Neufchâtel)
5 sesame melba toast rounds
2 tablespoons finely chopped seedless cucumber
1 tablespoon finely chopped red onion
1/2 ounce thinly sliced smoked salmon, cut into strips

Spread the cheese on the toast rounds. Top with the cucumber, onion, and salmon.

■ **PER SERVING (5 TOASTS):** 120 calories, 4 g total fat, 2 g saturated fat, 14 mg cholesterol, 265 mg sodium, 14 g total carbohydrates, 1 g dietary fiber, 6 g protein, 20 mg calcium ■ *POINTS PER SERVING: 3*


# Crunchy Zucchini Sticks

This cornflake coating also works well on other vegetables. Try making crunchy mushroom caps or onion rings, if you like.

### MAKES 6 SERVINGS

1 zucchini, cut into 4 × 1/2-inch sticks (about 24)
1 yellow squash, cut into 4 × 1/2-inch sticks (about 24)
2 tablespoons reduced-calorie mayonnaise
6 tablespoons cornflake crumbs

Preheat the broiler. Spray a large baking sheet with nonstick spray. Combine the zucchini, yellow squash and mayonnaise in a bowl until well coated. Place the cornflake crumbs in a zip-close plastic bag. Add the zucchini and yellow squash in batches, shaking the bag to coat both sides. Arrange the vegetables in one layer on the baking sheet. Spray the top of the vegetables lightly with nonstick spray. Broil 7 inches from the heat until the vegetables are tender and golden, about 3 minutes on each side.

■ PER SERVING (8 STICKS): 40 calories, 2 g total fat, 0 g saturated fat, 2 mg cholesterol, 69 mg sodium, 5 g total carbohydrates, 1 g dietary fiber, 1 g protein, 10 mg calcium ■ *POINTS PER SERVING: 1*

# Cheddar Crisps

L ike an open-face quesadilla, these cheddar crisps make a tasty snack in minutes. They are also delicious when served as a party appetizer.

MAKES 4 SERVINGS

1/2 cup shredded reduced-fat cheddar cheese
2 tablespoons grated Parmesan cheese
1/8 teaspoon cayenne
2 (6-inch) fat-free flour tortillas

Preheat the oven to 450° F. Spray a baking sheet with nonstick spray. Combine the cheddar cheese, Parmesan cheese, and cayenne in a small bowl. Place the tortillas on the baking sheet and top with the cheese mixture. Bake until the tortillas are crisp and the cheese is melted, about 8 minutes. Cut the tortillas in fourths, making a total of 8 pieces.

■ PER SERVING (2 CRISPS): 85 calories, 3 g total fat, 2 g saturated fat, 10 mg cholesterol, 189 mg sodium, 7 g total carbohydrates, 0 g dietary fiber, 6 g protein, 161 mg calcium ■ *POINTS PER SERVING: 2*

# Maple Granola Bars

These portable, high-energy bars are an excellent addition to school lunches, picnics, or car trips. For a special treat, drizzle the cooled cookies with a little melted chocolate.

MAKES 10 SERVINGS

3 cups quick-cooking rolled oats
1 cup raisins, chopped
1/2 cup sliced almonds, chopped
1 teaspoon ground cinnamon
1/2 teaspoon salt
1/4 cup maple syrup
1/4 cup honey
1/4 cup water
1 tablespoon packed dark brown sugar

1. Preheat the oven to 325° F. Spray a baking sheet with nonstick spray.
2. Combine the oats, raisins, almonds, cinnamon, and salt in a large bowl.
3. Bring the syrup, honey, water, and brown sugar to a boil in a small saucepan; remove from the heat. Pour over the oat mixture, stirring well to coat. With wet hands, shape the mixture into ten 4-inch logs. Place the logs on the baking sheet and flatten to 1/2-inch thickness.
4. Bake until the bars are slightly firm to the touch, about 30 minutes. Cool on the baking sheet 5 minutes; remove from the baking sheet and cool completely on a rack. Store the granola bars in an airtight container.

■ PER SERVING (1 BAR): 220 calories, 4 g total fat, 1 g saturated fat, 0 mg cholesterol, 122 mg sodium, 43 g total carbohydrates, 4 g dietary fiber, 5 g protein, 45 mg calcium ■ *POINTS PER SERVING: 4*

# Cinnamon-Sugar Popcorn

≡

**H**ere is a three-ingredient pick-me-up the whole family will love.

MAKES 8 SERVINGS

8 cups plain, hot-air-popped popcorn
2 tablespoons superfine sugar
1 tablespoon ground cinnamon

Place the popcorn in a large bowl. Lightly spray with butter-flavored nonstick spray. Add the sugar and cinnamon; toss to coat.

■ **PER SERVING (1 CUP):** 45 calories, 0 g total fat, 0 g saturated fat, 0 mg cholesterol, 1 mg sodium, 10 g total carbohydrates, 2 g dietary fiber, 1 g protein, 11 mg calcium ■ *POINTS PER SERVING: 1*

# Peanut Butter and Banana Rice Cakes

≡

**R**ice cakes make a low-calorie, crunchy alternative to bread.

MAKES 4 SERVINGS

2 tablespoons semisweet chocolate chips, melted
4 multigrain rice cakes
2 tablespoons reduced-fat peanut butter
1 banana, sliced
4 teaspoons honey

Divide the melted chocolate evenly over the rice cakes. Refrigerate 5 minutes to allow the chocolate to harden. Top each rice cake with the peanut butter and banana. Drizzle 1 teaspoon of the honey over each cake. Serve at once.

■ **PER SERVING (1 RICE CAKE):** 139 calories, 5 g total fat, 1 g saturated fat, 0 mg cholesterol, 81 mg sodium, 22 g total carbohydrates, 2 g dietary fiber, 4 g protein, 10 mg calcium ■ *POINTS PER SERVING: 3*

# Quick-Fix Yogurt Parfait

MAKES 1 SERVING

1 cup nonfat peach yogurt
1 cup peach slices, blueberries, or raspberries
2 tablespoons low-fat granola
Freshly grated nutmeg

Layer the yogurt, fruit, and granola in a parfait glass. Sprinkle with the nutmeg.

■ PER SERVING (1 PARFAIT): 274 calories, 1 g total fat, 0 g saturated fat, 5 mg cholesterol, 103 mg sodium, 58 g total carbohydrates, 4 g dietary fiber, 12 g protein, 337 mg calcium ■ *POINTS PER SERVING: 5*

# Papaya Smoothie

This smoothie keeps well in the refrigerator for up to 3 days. Serve with fresh mint.

MAKES 2 SERVINGS (3 CUPS)

1 papaya, halved and seeds removed
2 kiwi fruits, halved
1 cup orange juice
4 teaspoons honey
2 teaspoons fresh lime or lemon juice
8 ice cubes

Scoop the papaya flesh and the kiwi fruit flesh into a blender. Add the orange juice, honey, and lime or lemon juice; pulse until smooth. Add the ice cubes and pulse until slightly crushed.

■ PER SERVING (1 1/2 CUPS): 205 calories, 1 g total fat, 0 g saturated fat, 0 mg cholesterol, 12 mg sodium, 52 g total carbohydrates, 6 g dietary fiber, 3 g protein, 70 mg calcium ■ *POINTS PER SERVING: 3*

# Recommended Reading

Albert, Katherine A. *Get a Good Night's Sleep.* New York: Simon & Schuster, 1996.

Atkinson, Holly. *Women and Fatigue.* New York: Pocket Books, 1987.

Benson, Herbert. *The Relaxation Response.* New York: HarperTorch, 2000.

Burns, David D. *The Feeling Good Handbook.* New York: Plume, 1999.

Domar, Alice, and Henry Dreher. *Self-Nurture: Learning to Care for Yourself as Effectively as You Care for Everyone Else.* New York: Viking, 2000.

Johnson, Karen. *Trusting Ourselves: The Complete Guide to Emotional Well-Being for Women.* New York: Atlantic Monthly Press, 1991.

Kabat-Zinn, Jon. *Wherever You Go, There You Are: Mindfulness Meditation in Everyday Life.* New York: Hyperion, 1994.

Kirby, Jane. *Dieting for Dummies.* Foster City, Calif.: IDG Books, 1998.

Lamberg, Lynne. *Bodyrhythms: Chronobiology and Peak Performance.* New York: William Morrow and Company, 1994.

Ravicz, Simone. *High on Stress: A Woman's Guide to Optimizing the Stress in Her Life.* Oakland, Calif.: New Harbinger Publications, 1998.

Somer, Elizabeth. *Food & Mood: The Complete Guide to Eating Well and Feeling Your Best.* New York: Henry Holt and Company, 1995.

Thayer, Robert E. *The Origin of Everyday Moods: Managing Energy, Tension, and Stress.* New York: Oxford University Press, 1996.

# Index